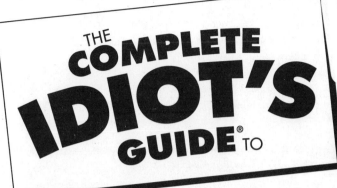
THE COMPLETE **IDIOT'S** GUIDE® TO

Arthritis

by Amye L. Leong, M.B.A.,
Neal S. Birnbaum, M.D., FACP, FACR, and
Karen K. Brees, Ph.D.

ALPHA

A member of Penguin Group (USA) Inc.

We dedicate this book to the empowerment of people affected by arthritis.

ALPHA BOOKS

Published by the Penguin Group

Penguin Group (USA) Inc., 375 Hudson Street, New York, New York 10014, USA

Penguin Group (Canada), 90 Eglinton Avenue East, Suite 700, Toronto, Ontario M4P 2Y3, Canada (a division of Pearson Penguin Canada Inc.)

Penguin Books Ltd., 80 Strand, London WC2R 0RL, England

Penguin Ireland, 25 St. Stephen's Green, Dublin 2, Ireland (a division of Penguin Books Ltd.)

Penguin Group (Australia), 250 Camberwell Road, Camberwell, Victoria 3124, Australia (a division of Pearson Australia Group Pty. Ltd.)

Penguin Books India Pvt. Ltd., 11 Community Centre, Panchsheel Park, New Delhi—110 017, India

Penguin Group (NZ), 67 Apollo Drive, Rosedale, North Shore, Auckland 1311, New Zealand (a division of Pearson New Zealand Ltd.)

Penguin Books (South Africa) (Pty.) Ltd., 24 Sturdee Avenue, Rosebank, Johannesburg 2196, South Africa

Penguin Books Ltd., Registered Offices: 80 Strand, London WC2R 0RL, England

International Standard Book Number: 978-1-59257-837-5
Library of Congress Catalog Card Number: 2008937770

11 10 09   8 7 6 5 4 3 2 1

Interpretation of the printing code: The rightmost number of the first series of numbers is the year of the book's printing; the rightmost number of the second series of numbers is the number of the book's printing. For example, a printing code of 09-1 shows that the first printing occurred in 2009.

Printed in the United States of America

Note: This publication contains the opinions and ideas of its authors. It is intended to provide helpful and informative material on the subject matter covered. It is sold with the understanding that the authors and publisher are not engaged in rendering professional services in the book. If the reader requires personal assistance or advice, a competent professional should be consulted.

The authors and publisher specifically disclaim any responsibility for any liability, loss, or risk, personal or otherwise, which is incurred as a consequence, directly or indirectly, of the use and application of any of the contents of this book.

Most Alpha books are available at special quantity discounts for bulk purchases for sales promotions, premiums, fund-raising, or educational use. Special books, or book excerpts, can also be created to fit specific needs.

For details, write: Special Markets, Alpha Books, 375 Hudson Street, New York, NY 10014.

Publisher: *Marie Butler-Knight*
Editorial Director: *Mike Sanders*
Senior Managing Editor: *Billy Fields*
Senior Acquisitions Editor: *Paul Dinas*
Development Editor: *Lynn Northrup*
Senior Production Editor: *Janette Lynn*
Copy Editor: *Teresa Elsey*

Cover Designer: *William Thomas*
Book Designer: *Trina Wurst*
Cartoonist: *Steve Barr*
Indexer: *Angie Bess*
Layout: *Ayanna Lacey*
Proofreader: *John Etchison*

Contents at a Glance

Appendixes

Contents

Appendixes

Introduction

Arthritis affects nearly 46 million Americans—almost 300,000 of them children—and countless millions more worldwide. From the wear and tear on joints that results in osteoarthritis to the malfunction of the body's immune system that leads to rheumatoid arthritis and other forms of inflammatory arthritis, this disease touches all of us.

The word *arthritis* means inflammation of the joints, but that's just touching the surface. Arthritis causes pain, stiffness, swollen joints, and in some cases, serious disability. There is no cure for arthritis yet, but we can treat its symptoms. Recent discoveries of new medications have improved the quality of life for many people with serious forms of arthritis. In some cases, the results have been nothing short of miraculous. Still, there is much work to be done if we are to find the cure.

Living well with arthritis means taking an active role in your health care. That means watching your diet, combining exercise with rest, conserving your energy whenever possible, and using the resources available to you. It also means educating yourself about arthritis, seeking professional guidance and treatment from the health-care professionals who are knowledgeable about arthritis, and following their recommendations.

Arthritis used to be thought of as a disease of old people. We know now that's not true. Arthritis can affect young children, teenagers, young adults, and the middle-aged, as well as the elderly. It doesn't discriminate on the basis of age, gender, ethnicity, or race. We are all vulnerable, but that vulnerability has heightened our awareness and fueled our desire to find the cure.

Each day the cure gets closer. You can add your voice and your support to the cause. Support legislation that funds research by writing to your state legislators. Make your wishes known. Join the Arthritis Foundation and become part of the future. Think you're just one person and that you won't have any effect? In the words of Margaret Mead, American anthropologist: "Never doubt that a small group of thoughtful, committed citizens can change the world. Indeed, it's the only thing that ever has."

How to Use This Book

This book is a ready reference for anyone interested in learning more about arthritis—its causes, symptoms, and treatment. Read the general information and then find the chapter or chapters that answer your specific questions. It's divided into four parts:

Part 1, "Understanding Arthritis," explains how healthy joints work and what happens when arthritis enters the picture. You'll learn to recognize the symptoms of arthritis and how to navigate your first appointment with your rheumatologist.

Part 2, "The Different Types of Arthritis," gives you an overview of some of the most common forms of arthritis, along with explanations of symptoms, causes and risk factors, diagnosis, and treatment.

Part 3, "The Path to Treatment," takes the next step after diagnosis. You'll learn about various treatment options: medications, lifestyle changes, surgery, and complementary medicine.

Part 4, "Living with Arthritis," gives you helpful information on managing pain, fighting fatigue, maintaining your family life, and managing your work life.

You'll also find three appendixes: a glossary that defines unfamiliar terms, a handy list of acronyms, and resources for further information.

Extras

You'll find all kinds of tidbits of useful information scattered throughout the book. Look for these pearls of wisdom:

Consultation

The doctor is in! Here's sage advice free of charge.

Precautions

Check these boxes for cautions you need to be aware of.

Straight Talk

In these boxes you'll find timely advice and helpful words from real people with arthritis.

def•i•ni•tion

Some medical terms defy translation! Here's the breakdown in simple English.

Acknowledgments

No one is responsible for my getting three different forms of crippling arthritis, but rising up out of a wheelchair to become an international patient advocate took the love and persistence of family and friends, and even innocent bystanders. First, my parents, Harvey and Jeanne Leong, and sister Christine, looked beyond our Chinese culture of disability and shame to provide me the love and facility to get through each day of pain. I realize that extra attention demanded by the disease of my parents for my medical care took away from that of my sister, so I am grateful to have a big sister we all call "J" (Jay-Jay means big sister in Chinese) to always be there when I needed a big sister. Love goes to my niece, Amye Michelle Chow, and nephews, Christopher and Nicholas Chow, who grew up seeing their auntie in hospitals and playing with the arthritis-friendly gadgets as a normal part of their everyday life, who have become wonderful young adults today sensitive to the needs of anyone in pain.

My thanks to the thousands of people I've met through speaking engagements around the U.S.A. and in 15 countries who heard my stories of determination. They not only walked away inspired to make their own arthritis battle one of emotional victory over physical disease, but also became determined to work with their physicians to achieve acceptable success and transformed themselves into personal patient advocates. I thank the establishment of physicians and health professionals who, back in the early 1980s, took a chance to let me into the inner circle of professional associations despite my not having the appropriate letters after my name. Today, patient advocates are an integrated force, indeed a movement of caring, eloquent, and effective people who speak up for our physicians in crises because there's not enough trained rheumatologists to care for the millions in need. I am honored to have broken physician-patient barriers for so many other advocate colleagues today.

And finally, to the innocent bystanders who tilted their heads and furrowed their brows in rejection of seeing a crippled me trying to hobble across the street before the light turned red, I say "thank you." Your questionable looks of disbelief motivated me to spring out of the doldrums of physical and emotional disability to educate myself and fight for the services I needed to regain my independence. Those bystanders motivated me to understand the power of my own will and intellect in dealing effectively with arthritis. If I can do it, you can too. Go for it!

—Amye L. Leong, M.B.A.

I need to thank Linda, my wife of 37 years, for not only tolerating but supporting all the evenings and weekends away from family while I've pursued my professional career. I'm also grateful to the late Dr. Gerald Rodnan, who ignited my interest in rheumatology at the University of Pittsburgh in 1973.

—Neal S. Birnbaum, M.D., FACP, FACR

I would like to thank Andrea Hurst, agent *par excellence*, Paul Dinas, senior acquisitions editor for Alpha Books, Lynn Northrup, development editor for Alpha Books, and Janette Lynn, senior production editor for Alpha Books.

—Karen K. Brees, Ph.D.

Trademarks

All terms mentioned in this book that are known to be or are suspected of being trademarks or service marks have been appropriately capitalized. Alpha Books and Penguin Group (USA) Inc. cannot attest to the accuracy of this information. Use of a term in this book should not be regarded as affecting the validity of any trademark or service mark.

Part 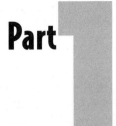1

Understanding Arthritis

Arthritis is not a single disease, nor is it just a disease that affects the elderly. Arthritis is a broad term, encompassing more than 100 rheumatic diseases. Nearly 46 million Americans suffer from arthritis and related conditions. More than 8.3 million are young adults and about 294,000 are children.

In Part 1, we'll take an in-depth look at just what arthritis is and how it impacts joint function and, in some cases, major organs as well. We'll examine risk factors that may predispose you to develop arthritis and show you how to use a symptom log to help you decide when it's time to see the doctor.

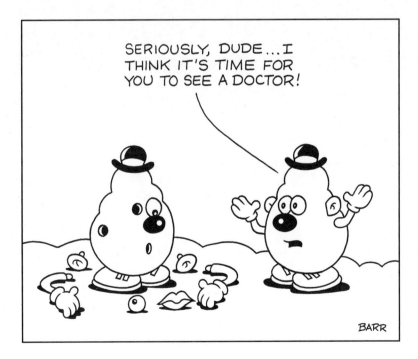

Chapter 1

Arthritis: What It Is and What It Does

In This Chapter

- Understanding what arthritis is
- Anyone can get arthritis
- Myths and misconceptions
- The financial cost of arthritis
- Are you at risk?

Arthritis, in its broadest sense, means "inflammation of the joints." Your joints are designed to move freely, but when arthritis enters the picture, that free movement becomes difficult and often painful. There are many myths surrounding the causes and treatment of arthritis. Knowing what's true and what's not can save you time, money, and unnecessary discomfort.

What Is Arthritis?

When you hear people talk about arthritis, it may seem as if they're referring to a single disease, but this isn't accurate. *Arthritis* is a common term used to cover a group of more than 100 different *rheumatic diseases* affecting nearly 46 million adults and 300,000 children in the United States. Countless millions worldwide are also affected. Osteoarthritis is the most common form of arthritis in the United States, followed by gout, fibromyalgia, and rheumatoid arthritis.

def•i•ni•tion

A **rheumatic disease** is a disease that causes inflammation of the body's connective tissues, especially the joints (the places where two or more bones meet).

You may have occasionally heard arthritis referred to as *rheumatism*. This is an older term used to describe disorders that cause aches and pains and involve muscles, joints, bones, and tendons. In fact, back in 1931, Gene Autry recorded "The Rheumatism Blues," a song complaining about his rheumatism.

Today we know that these disorders have different symptoms, different causes, and different treatments, and so we refer to them by their specific names—rheumatoid arthritis, gouty arthritis, osteoarthritis, lupus (systemic lupus erythematosus)—instead of lumping them into one general category.

There are two major categories of arthritis. The first category involves arthritis caused by wear and tear on your body's joints. It can be a product of the aging process, be caused by injury, or be the eventual outcome of repetitive motion that causes a joint to wear out. This type of arthritis is called *degenerative arthritis* or *osteoarthritis*.

The second category concerns conditions that are inflammatory and sometimes systemic, meaning they can affect any part of your body, including organs such as the heart, lungs, and kidneys. These types of arthritis may develop as a result of malfunctions in the body's immune system. The causes of these types of arthritis are being studied by researchers, and many factors may play a role. Rheumatoid arthritis is one type of inflammatory arthritis.

Arthritis is a chronic disease. This means that symptoms can come and go but generally last over a long period of time. It's also possible to have more than one form of arthritis at the same time.

Regardless of the type of arthritis you have, early diagnosis and treatment are key to managing it. Medication, exercise balanced with rest, maintaining a proper weight, and surgery—if it becomes necessary—are ways to treat arthritis. In order to understand what arthritis is and what it does, it's first important to know something about your joints—how they're designed and how they work.

How Healthy Joints Function

Healthy joints are marvels of design and engineering. They allow flexibility along with stability. They support your weight. They allow you to move with grace and skill, tie your shoes, brush your teeth, engage in sports, play a musical instrument, walk, skip, jump, run, and dance. In short, if it involves movement, it involves a joint, which is simply the place where two bones meet.

Your body has different types of joints that have different kinds of movements and functions. Some joints, such as the ones in your skull, are fixed—they don't move. Others are slightly movable, such as those between the vertebrae in your spine and your ribs; and still others move quite a bit, for example, your shoulders and hips and fingers.

Your joints rely on other structures to do their jobs. Ligaments connect the bones and keep joints stable. Muscles and tendons enable joints to move and give them power. The synovium and the cartilage are specific parts of your joints that allow them to function smoothly and without pain.

Consultation

The only bone in your body that doesn't form a joint with another bone is the hyoid bone, located in your neck. You have 206 bones in your body and over 360 joints. About 230 of these joints are moveable or semimovable.

The synovium is a membrane that lines the joint and produces fluid, called synovial fluid. Just as adding oil to a squeaky hinge allows the parts to function without grating against each other, synovial fluid lubricates the cartilage. It also delivers nutrients to it.

Cartilage is the rubbery, slippery tissue coating the ends of your bones and works like a shock absorber. Cartilage is one of the few tissues in the body that doesn't have its own blood supply, so it has to rely upon synovial fluid for its health.

In healthy joints, all of these parts work together to promote movement. When inflammation enters the picture, however, all this changes.

Explaining Inflammation

When you injure yourself, your body's immune system rushes to repair the damage. White blood cells are dispatched to the wound and certain chemical processes are set in motion. Inflammation is one of these processes. It's part of your body's arsenal of weapons against injury or infection. You notice that the skin around the injury gets red, feels warm to the touch, and may swell.

The process of inflammation is complex. Chemicals released by the body are responsible for the symptoms of inflammation. Some of these chemicals increase blood flow to the area that the body thinks is under attack. This results in the redness and warmth. Other chemicals cause fluid to leak into the tissues. This results in the swelling that you see. These chemicals can also stimulate nerve endings, causing pain.

Usually, once the injury has healed, everything returns to normal. Your skin cools, the redness goes away, and the swelling disappears. Sometimes, however, something goes wrong and the inflammation doesn't go away, but instead continues to act as if the injury still needs help recovering.

Sometimes the inflammatory process is triggered when there's no injury or infection to treat. It then actually attacks the body it's designed to protect! This malfunction of the immune system then becomes an autoimmune disease. Certain types of arthritis, such as rheumatoid arthritis (RA) and systemic lupus erythematosus (SLE)—commonly referred to as lupus—are autoimmune diseases, caused by an immune system that's gone haywire.

Eventually, this oversupply of white blood cells, chemicals, and inflammation can create irritation, damage the body's cartilage, and cause the pain and stiffness that you are experiencing. Inflammation comes with many symptoms, although not all of them may be present at the same time.

Your joint may be red and swollen. It may hurt to touch it and there can be pain. You may also notice it's difficult to use that joint.

Sometimes, inflammation may feel like the flu, and you may find yourself experiencing all the symptoms you'd associated with it, such as chills and fever, headache, fatigue, and generally feeling lousy all over.

Symptoms can develop gradually over time or come on suddenly. The pattern and location of the symptoms you experience will be uniquely your own, which can make diagnosis difficult.

Precautions

Pain doesn't have to be present for you to have arthritis. When arthritis is part of a systemic problem, the systemic illness may affect an organ that doesn't have many pain-sensitive nerves. When you're experiencing any symptoms of arthritis, prompt diagnosis and treatment are important to prevent organ damage.

You may find that you're dealing with a collection of symptoms that don't seem to indicate anything specific, but your physician will put everything together and make the proper diagnosis. That's why it's important to talk to your doctor if you're experiencing a rash of symptoms that aren't going away.

Who Gets Arthritis?

The answer is *anyone*. Anyone can develop arthritis at any time. Arthritis doesn't play favorites. It's no respecter of age, gender, or ethnic background. In fact, arthritis has been around since the time of the dinosaurs, and these early creatures were early victims of arthritis. Fossilized remains of a herd of iguanodons, which roamed in the vicinity of what is now Brussels, Belgium, about 85 million years ago, show evidence of ankle osteoarthritis!

Once the dinos were gone, arthritis introduced itself to the Neanderthals, distant relatives of modern man who lived about 30,000 years ago. Anthropologists have discovered that Neanderthals suffered from osteoarthritis—probably resulting from injuries or from the harsh realities of their daily existence. Interestingly enough, these are some of the same reasons we develop osteoarthritis today.

Evidence of arthritis in humans dates back to 4500 B.C.E. It was found in the skeletal remains of Native Americans who lived in what are now Tennessee and Olathe, Kansas. And halfway around the Earth, 2,000 years later, the Egyptians also had to deal with arthritis, as evidenced by X-rays of their mummies.

Historical figures closer to modern times weren't exempt either. King Henry VIII of England, Leonardo da Vinci, Auguste Renoir, and Benjamin Franklin led very different lives but had arthritis in common.

Consultation

The famous Ötzi the Iceman mummy that was found in the Alps near the border of Italy and Austria also had arthritis. He lived and died around 3000 B.C.E. and, judging from the package of medicinal herbs he was carrying, perhaps he was trying to do something about his symptoms.

Today, according to the Centers for Disease Control and Prevention (CDC), 294,000 children under age 18 in the United States have arthritis—that breaks down to about 1 in every 250 children. And as you age, your chances of developing arthritis increase.

Of persons aged 18–44, almost 8 percent (8.7 million) report doctor-diagnosed arthritis. Of persons aged 45–64, over 29 percent (20.5 million) report doctor-diagnosed arthritis. Of persons aged 65 and older, 50 percent (17.2 million) report doctor-diagnosed arthritis. As the baby boomer generation ages, these numbers will swell. It is projected that by 2030, 67 million Americans aged 18 years or older will have been diagnosed with arthritis.

Separating Fact from Fiction

There are many myths and misconceptions associated with arthritis and they run the gamut from risk factors to sure cures. Want to cure arthritis? Put some potatoes in your pocket. It sounds silly now, but that old wives' tale lasted for quite some time. It may have been that a pocketful of potatoes was so uncomfortable that the discomfort was greater than your stiff knee. Other myths are still around:

- **Arthritis is a disease of old people.** It's true that your risk for arthritis—especially osteoarthritis—increases as you age, but it's also true that nearly three out of five people with arthritis are younger than 65. Juvenile arthritis is one of the most common chronic childhood diseases. Arthritis can affect any one of any age.

- **Arthritis is a normal part of the aging process.** If that were true, children wouldn't get arthritis—but they do. Arthritis that develops as an autoimmune disease, such as rheumatoid arthritis, is not part of normal aging.

- **There's nothing you can do to prevent the worsening of arthritis.** Wrong. Osteoarthritis can often be slowed by lifestyle changes, such as losing excess weight and balancing rest with exercise.

- **Arthritis isn't serious.** Wrong again. Arthritis is the number-one cause of disability in the United States.

- **Cold, damp weather causes arthritis.** Not true, although research is showing that cold and damp can aggravate symptoms of arthritis that are already there.

- **Eating foods from the nightshade family (tomatoes and potatoes) will make rheumatoid arthritis worse.** There's no truth in this one. No research confirms the link between specific foods and arthritis.

- **Knuckle-cracking causes arthritis.** Nope. It's merely an annoying habit.

- **Wearing a copper bracelet will cure arthritis.** Nope again. As a fashion statement, it can tell the world you have arthritis, however.

Myths tend to hang on long after research has proven them to be inaccurate. Once something gets ingrained in folklore, it's got staying power.

The Financial Impact of Arthritis

Adding up the total financial impact of arthritis is no easy task. The Centers for Disease Control (CDC) reports that in 2003, the total cost attributed to arthritis and other rheumatic conditions in the United States was $128 billion, up from $86.2 billion in 1997. These figures include direct and indirect costs but don't take into account the amount of money people spend on unproven remedies—a figure estimated to be almost $2 billion annually.

This amount is guaranteed to increase dramatically as our population ages. There are obvious direct costs related to the diagnosis and treatment of arthritis, such as doctor fees, hospital costs, medications, and therapy, but the associated costs are the real budget breakers.

As reported in the journal *Arthritis and Rheumatism* (2007), the Medical Expenditures Panel Study looked at a sample of households across the country in which arthritis and related rheumatic conditions were present. They totaled up the costs of medical care plus individual loss of income for those participating in the study.

They found that expenditures for arthritis medications nearly doubled between 1997 and 2003. The mean number of prescriptions per patient jumped from 18.7 to 25.2 and the mean cost of a prescription rose from $48 to $65. Inpatient hospital costs declined from $508 to $352 per person over the same period. This meant that overall, expenditures remained fairly stable.

Where there was a significant increase, however, was in loss of earnings. In 1997, loss of earnings for employed people with arthritis or another rheumatic condition was about $99 billion. In 2003, that number rose to $108 billion.

The researchers concluded that these numbers would continue to rise, since the number of people with arthritis and other rheumatic conditions is expected to steadily increase.

According to the Arthritis Foundation, less than half of rheumatoid arthritis patients under 65 years old who are working at the onset of the disease are still working 10 years later. The journal *Arthritis and Rheumatism* (2004) reported that among adults with doctor-diagnosed arthritis, many reported significant limitations in vital activities such as ...

- Walking one quarter mile (6 million).
- Stooping, bending, and kneeling (7.8 million).

♦ Climbing stairs (4.8 million).

♦ Participating in social activities such as church and family gatherings (2.1 million).

According to the CDC, total costs attributable to arthritis and other rheumatic conditions in the United States in 2003 equaled 1.2 percent of the 2003 U.S. gross domestic product.

Arthritis can have a broad impact on all areas of life, from loss of income resulting from missed work days to disability resulting in loss of employment. It's a serious concern.

Risk Factors for Arthritis

As with many other medical conditions, there are risk factors for arthritis that are beyond your control and risk factors over which you have a great deal of control. Here's a rundown of factors you can control, factors you may have some influence over, and factors that you can't do much about.

Consultation

The National Center for Chronic Disease Promotion, an agency of the CDC, reports that 66 percent of adults with doctor-diagnosed arthritis are overweight or obese, as compared to 53 percent of adults without doctor-diagnosed arthritis.

Are you overweight? Being overweight stresses your knees and hips and is known to increase your chances of developing osteoarthritis (OA) of the knee and hip. Losing as little as 11 pounds reduces the risk of developing knee osteoarthritis among women by 50 percent.

Throughout history, fashion and common sense have not usually been on good terms with each other. Some of fashion's more extreme styles, in fact, can create all kinds of insults to the human body, but the millions of dollars spent on advertising can often sway even the most sensible person.

If you are a woman, do you wear high heels? One study investigated how much force was transferred to the leg joints of 20 women who wore high heels. Participants walked barefoot and then put on their shoes. Measurements indicated greater force across both the knee and hip joints, along with an average of 23 percent more force to the leg joints, when women walked in their heels.

Why is this important? Excessive force on the knee caused by wearing heels may contribute to degenerative changes in the knee joint and other leg joints. Since osteoarthritis (OA) of the knee is twice as common in women as in men, high heels may be part of the problem.

Do you smoke? The percentage of people who smoke has decreased by nearly 50 percent over the past 20 years, but if you're among the percentage who still do, you're putting yourself at increased risk for a variety of medical conditions, including arthritis.

> **Straight Talk**
>
> People have been sacrificing their health for fashion since time immemorial: "All this I see; and I see that the fashion wears out more apparel than the man."
>
> —Shakespeare, *Much Ado About Nothing*

According to a study published in *Annals of the Rheumatic Diseases* (1997), smoking may influence the development and severity of arthritis. For this study, researchers used questionnaires to examine the cigarette smoking history and habits of people who had had a complete physical examination and had been found to have arthritis.

They found strong evidence of a link between cigarette smoking and rheumatoid arthritis. Smokers who reported at least 25 "pack years" (a certain number of packs of cigarettes smoked equaled one pack year) were more likely to display symptoms of arthritis, including swollen or tender joints, and factors contributing to the development of rheumatoid arthritis. Rheumatoid arthritis appears to be both more common and more severe in smokers than nonsmokers. Yet another reason not to smoke!

Some risk factors are within your ability to modify, but the modifications may require you to make significant changes. For example, if your line of work requires repetitive bending or kneeling, you may increase your chances of developing knee osteoarthritis. If you develop osteoarthritis, your symptoms may force you to change to an occupation that doesn't require you to use your affected joints.

If you participate in sports that have a high risk of injury to the joints, you may find that you develop osteoarthritis in your joints that have suffered injuries. For example, football players may injure their knees and then develop post-traumatic arthritis down the road.

Even if you are able to eliminate or at least reduce your risk factors in the areas over which you have some degree of control, there are certain risk factors that are beyond your ability to control. These include your age, your gender, and your genetics.

The risk of developing most types of arthritis increases with age. Most types of arthritis are more common in women; in fact, 60 percent of people with arthritis are women. Gout, however, is more common in men. Specific genes are associated with a higher risk of certain types of arthritis, such as rheumatoid arthritis (RA), systemic lupus erythematosus (SLE), and ankylosing spondylitis.

If you're a member of the baby boom generation, you belong to a group of about 77 million Americans who were born between 1946 and 1964, and you have now reached middle age. As part of a generation that has prided itself on remaining active, you may be discovering that your joints are beginning to show signs of wear and tear. Your knees, hips, spine, and other joints may not understand that you still feel young—they seem bent on reminding you about your chronological age! In fact, bending them may now be causing you considerable pain.

What else can bring on arthritis? You're probably familiar with strep infections and staph infections. Strep (*Streptococcus*) and staph (*Staphylococcus aureus*) are bacterial infections. They're also the most common causes of acute infectious arthritis.

These bacteria can access your body through a break or a cut in your skin or through an ear infection. Once inside, the bacteria travel through the bloodstream and settle in a joint, where the body's own defense system—the immune response—fights against the intruder. The end result is inflammation. If not treated promptly, severe joint damage can occur very quickly.

Another condition that's become well known in recent years is Lyme disease. Untreated Lyme disease, caused by a *spirochete* carried by the deer tick, can lead to infectious arthritis, as can untreated sexually transmitted diseases, particularly gonorrhea.

def•i•ni•tion

A **spirochete** is a microscopic bacterial organism. Spirochetes are spiral-shaped, sort of like worms. If you looked at one through a microscope, you'd be amazed at its high activity level.

Certain viruses can cause arthritic disorders to develop. One of these is parvovirus, which causes "fifth disease" or "slap cheek" in children (the latter term refers to the bright red cheeks in children with the virus). Parvovirus in adults can cause infectious arthritis to develop. If you contract parvovirus, symptoms often go away within a few weeks. However, occasionally the joint pain and swelling persist for up to one to two years. Symptoms in chronic parvovirus infection may closely mimic rheumatoid arthritis and may require similar treatment.

People with compromised immune systems may be at greater risk for developing infectious arthritis. If you have diabetes or sickle cell anemia, you may be among these at-risk individuals.

What can you do to protect yourself? The answers range from treating skin injuries with appropriate antibiotics to practicing safe sex to avoiding exposure to ticks that can carry Lyme disease. (See Chapter 8 for more on Lyme disease.)

If you're leading an active lifestyle, you're not going to let your chronological age dictate what kinds of sports or leisure-time activities you'll enjoy. But there's a price to be paid for all of our biking, tennis playing, basketball pickup games, and softball league participation.

According to the American Academy of Orthopaedic Surgeons, about 4.1 million people seek medical care for knee problems each year. In 2005, 498,169 total knee replacements were performed. If you want to continue playing and enjoying life, follow some of their recommendations:

- ◆ Always warm up before beginning a sports activity. Do some sustained muscle stretching and spend three to five minutes warming up on a stationary bicycle or jogging.

- ◆ Don't skimp on your equipment. Good-quality shoes designed for the specific sport you are playing are essential.

- ◆ Make exercise part of your daily routine. A half hour of daily exercise will keep you in good shape. If you're just a weekend warrior, don't expect to go full out on the weekends and not pay the price afterward.

- ◆ Use the 10 percent rule as a guide when you want to increase your activity level. Up your intensity or repetitions by no more than 10 percent to avoid putting your joints under extreme stress. For example, go from shooting baskets for 50 minutes to shooting baskets for 55 minutes or from running a mile to running 1.1 miles.

- ◆ Alternate strength training with aerobic activity.

- ◆ Maintain a reasonable weight. Extra weight puts more stress on your knees.

- ◆ Don't overdo it. Listen to your body. When you feel that it's time to stop an activity, it probably is.

Injuries can be serious at any age, but they can be especially serious as we age. Take care of your joints and they'll last longer!

The Least You Need to Know

♦ *Arthritis* is a term used to cover more than 100 different rheumatic diseases that affect nearly 46 million adults and 300,000 children in the United States.

♦ Osteoarthritis, the most common form of arthritis in the United States, results from wear and tear on your body's joints.

♦ Anyone can get arthritis, regardless of age, gender, or ethnic background.

♦ Get the facts from your doctor. Don't rely on myths to manage your arthritis.

♦ The financial impact of arthritis is enormous and increasing exponentially.

♦ You can reduce your risk of certain types of arthritis through lifestyle changes and good health practices.

Chapter 2

Could It Be Arthritis?

In This Chapter

- ◆ Recognizing the symptoms of arthritis
- ◆ Taking control
- ◆ Consultation and referral practices
- ◆ Staffing your health-care team

Not every ache and pain is arthritis or part of an arthritis-related condition, but when those discomforts are signs of a larger problem, you need to know what to do about them. Early diagnosis can make a world of difference in how you feel and your enjoyment of life. While most forms of arthritis are not curable, almost everyone can be treated to either reduce or completely control their symptoms, and hopefully to slow or halt them from getting worse.

The first step is arriving at an accurate diagnosis. After this happens, you'll begin your treatment plan, which may consist of medications, lifestyle changes, and perhaps surgery. All along the way you'll be helped by the members of your health-care team.

Sorting Through the Symptoms

Over 100 rheumatologic conditions can cause joint pain or arthritis. The common symptoms of arthritis can also be associated with other medical conditions. Generally speaking, pain, stiffness, and sometimes swelling in your joints are the hallmark symptoms. The pain will be aggravated when you use the joint that is affected. For example, if you have knee osteoarthritis, walking can be painful. If you have rheumatoid arthritis, grasping items with your hands may become difficult or even impossible.

Only your doctor is qualified to make a definitive diagnosis of arthritis, and the process can take some time. She'll begin by listening to you explain your symptoms and performing a physical examination. Specific laboratory tests and X-rays of your affected joints will also help her in making a diagnosis.

Doing Your Homework

The patient-doctor relationship has undergone some transformations in recent years, and patients are now playing a larger part in managing their own health. Part of this is due to patients becoming more educated about their medical conditions, one of the benefits of the Information Age in which we live.

What this means for you is that it's in your best health interest to do your part to help your doctor help you. Becoming an educated consumer of health-care services will bring you many benefits, but to become that educated consumer, you'll need to be aware of what's going on with your body.

Keeping a Log

One day you wake up and feel stiff. It's probably not the first time you've felt this way, but this is the day you notice it and you realize it's like this every morning. There's a persistent pain in your hip. It comes and goes, but it's beginning to interfere with what you want to do and you find yourself pulling back from participating in activities that cause your hip to hurt.

Perhaps it's your hands. They're stiff, your knuckles seem to be swollen, and yesterday you couldn't pick up your toothbrush without a stab of pain. It's time to keep a log.

Logs don't have to be complex affairs. They're just a place where you jot down what you're feeling and when you're feeling it. Here are a couple of sample entries:

June 15

7:00 A.M. Right knee very stiff this morning. Difficult to bend it. Seemed better after I was up for a while. Continued to hurt throughout the morning.

June 16

8:30 A.M. Knee stiff again. Looks swollen and feels warm to the touch. Took some over-the-counter pain reliever. Seemed better later in the morning, but still hurts.

June 17

3:15 P.M. Tried to pick a book up from the table and felt a sharp pain. Had to drop the book.

As you can see, this is not Pulitzer Prize–winning writing, but it does the job. You're not trying to make your own diagnosis. You're compiling a record of your symptoms, so that you'll have something of substance to show the doctor when you make that appointment to get yourself checked out. Keep this journal for about two weeks. Then, if your symptoms are persisting, it's time to do something about them.

Consultation

How long should you wait before consulting a physician? The length of time depends upon your symptoms, of course. If your pain is intermittent, not too severe, and not interfering with your daily activities, such as with mild osteoarthritis, you may wait quite some time—months or even years. If your pain is acute, severe, and debilitating—such as with gout, which we'll discuss in Chapter 7—you need to seek help immediately.

Looking for Patterns

Symptoms come and go. That's true for many illnesses, and it's definitely true for arthritis. This can make a diagnosis difficult, and that's why medicine is an art as well as a science.

If you've noticed that your symptoms are worse in the morning, that's a pattern. If they're worse after you've been at an activity for a while, that's a pattern, too. Arriving at the proper diagnosis involves examining the patterns of your symptoms along with the characteristics of your symptoms. And that's why you'll need some professional medical help to get to the heart of the matter.

As you record your symptoms in your log, be sure to note the time of day and the activity you were engaged in when you felt pain or stiffness. This will be important information for your doctor.

Fears and Anxiety

Anytime things aren't going smoothly with your body, your concerns heighten. You wonder and fret and ask yourself all kinds of questions: Did I hurt myself? Is this the result of an injury? If these aches and pains are new to you, you may try to think back to when you might have injured the joint that is causing problems. You may be able to hone in on an event or you may come up short.

"Maybe if I just wait it will go away." That's an all-too-common response to physical symptoms that seem to arise from nowhere. It's probably not the best response if your symptoms last more than two weeks. Anything that lasts that long likely has an identifiable cause, and finding out what's causing your discomfort is important. If you do have arthritis, early diagnosis and treatment can make a world of difference in how you feel, so try not to ignore your symptoms. Instead, find out what's causing them. It just makes good sense.

"I know it's arthritis. Nothing can be done." Here you've made two errors. First, you've done a self-diagnosis, which is a risky venture. Second, you've jumped to a conclusion. It's time to take this problem to someone who has been trained in this area. It's time to consult your physician.

Two weeks is a very long time to endure pain. Remember, nobody is giving out medals for suffering. Besides, what if your doctor tells you that your condition can be treated and that treatment will allow you to get back into the swing of your daily life? Why wait? There's no magic number of days that declare "It's now time to talk to your doctor!" No, be smart. Gather your data, record it in your log, make an appointment with your physician, and begin getting back to the business of living.

Over-the-counter painkillers may offer temporary relief, but you want to know what's causing your symptoms. Then you can treat them properly. Of course you're concerned, but consulting your physician is the first step toward relieving that concern.

> **Consultation**
>
> It's a strange phenomenon. People sometimes think that if they go to the doctor they'll receive bad news. But ignoring your symptoms won't make them go away. Neither will postponing talking to your doctor. Making that appointment won't make your symptoms appear. Rather, you'll be taking positive steps to deal with them.

Begin at the Beginning

Make an appointment with your family health-care practitioner. He or she knows your medical history (if you've been getting an occasional complete physical examination) and will be more attuned to changes in your well-being.

Arthritis may appear with straightforward symptoms or it may be masked behind an array of vague discomforts. If you need a specialist, your physician will be able to refer you to a rheumatologist, a physician specializing in the treatment of arthritis and other rheumatic diseases.

A rheumatologist can make a definitive diagnosis of arthritis and also tell you what type of arthritis is causing your symptoms. If you have another rheumatologic disorder, your rheumatologist will be able to diagnose it and prescribe the appropriate treatment protocols for you.

Early Diagnosis Is Important

There are several reasons why early diagnosis is important. First of all, knowing what you're dealing with removes the doubt and concerns that cause stress to build. Second, if you've got osteoarthritis (OA)—the most common form of arthritis, which we'll cover in Chapter 3—beginning a treatment program early on will help slow the progress of the disease. For rheumatoid arthritis, early diagnosis is even more important, because early aggressive treatment can definitely slow or halt progression of joint damage.

Third, your symptoms may be caused by another condition altogether. Thinking you've got arthritis when you don't means a delay in getting appropriate treatment and can result in complications that could have been avoided. Finally, if you have one of the inflammatory kinds of arthritis, such as rheumatoid arthritis (RA), early intervention can reduce the chances of disability and joint deformity.

Precautions

Rheumatoid arthritis causes significant joint damage during the first two years after the symptoms of arthritis appear. Waiting for a diagnosis is not good medicine!

Appointments and Referrals

As you've already seen, arriving at a correct diagnosis can take some time and considerable expertise. Your family health-care practitioner may refer you to a rheumatologist.

A week or so before the date of your rheumatology appointment, call to be sure they have received the referral from your primary-care physician. Also, if your doctor took X-rays or performed any other diagnostic tests, check to see if the results have been received. If they haven't arrived, call your primary doctor's office to follow up. This will save time at your rheumatology appointment.

What should you take to that first rheumatology appointment? Your symptom log, for starters. Everyone's pattern of symptoms is unique, and that log will be immensely helpful for your rheumatologist in making the correct diagnosis. Be sure it's up-to-date. Also bring a picture ID. Many practices now record your picture with your file.

Consultation

Check with your insurance carrier for their requirements regarding referrals to specialists. Ultimately it is your responsibility to be sure their protocols, such as a written referral to a specialist or a prior authorization from the insurer, have been followed in order to avoid delays in payment of fees.

You'll also want to bring information regarding your past surgeries (including dates) and major illnesses and a list of all medications you are currently taking, along with their dosages. Remember to include all over-the-counter drugs, and also list any medications you're allergic to. Finally, bring a list of your questions. Don't expect to rely on memory at this point. Having them written down ahead of time will ensure that you don't forget anything important.

Meeting Your Rheumatologist

Plan to arrive 15–30 minutes before your scheduled appointment to allow time to go through the registration and check-in procedures. You'll be given a stack of papers to fill out (if they weren't sent to you in advance), regarding your medical history and insurance coverage. You will sign a form regarding privacy issues. This form allows your physicians to share information with each other about your condition.

After returning the completed forms, you'll be entered into the office's computer files. Once that's done, you'll be ready to meet the doctor. Expect this first appointment to involve a great deal of conversation. Your doctor will have questions, and, since you're prepared with your list, you'll have questions, too. If you don't understand the answers to your questions, ask for clarification. It's essential that you understand everything your doctor is saying.

Avoid the trap of agreeing with your doctor just to be, well, agreeable. If you're hearing something that doesn't jibe with what you're experiencing, say so. It's also essential to be truthful. Don't minimize your symptoms and don't exaggerate them either. In order to get the best care, you've got to be straightforward with your rheumatologist. Being honest with your doctor will build the foundation for a good doctor-patient relationship, one that's built upon mutual respect.

In some offices you'll first be seen by a nurse, nurse practitioner, or physician assistant. In others you'll see the rheumatologist right away.

What kinds of questions will the rheumatologist ask? Here's a list, so you can prepare!

- ◆ Where does it hurt? Is it just one joint or several joints?

- ◆ When does it hurt? When you use the joint or all the time?

- ◆ What does the pain feel like? Is it a dull aching pain, a sharp and stabbing one, or something else? What is your pain on a scale from 0 to 10?

- ◆ How long does your pain usually last? Does it come and go or is it constant?

- ◆ What aggravates the pain? What, if anything, provides you some relief?

- ◆ Does the pain interfere with your ability to perform any daily activities or tasks?

- ◆ Have you ever injured the joint that's bothering you?

- ◆ Recently, have you stressed or overused this joint? For example, have you done something out of the ordinary like spending an afternoon playing tennis or hiking?

- ◆ Do you have any other symptoms—rashes, fevers, weight loss, diarrhea, etc.?

- ◆ Does arthritis run in your family? Do you know what kind or kinds your family members have or had?

Answer these questions as completely as possible. This is where having your medical history with you will help immensely. Relying on your memory when you're stressed just makes you more stressed!

Consultation

Rheumatologists are some of the best medical detectives, and you may be puzzled by some of the questions you're asked that don't seem to relate to your symptoms. Why? Some types of arthritis develop after exposure to certain bacteria or viruses.

The Physical Examination

The physical examination will come next. At this time, the rheumatologist will be looking for visible evidence of arthritis. He'll examine your joints, and if any of them hurt during the exam, tell him. This is not the time to ignore your pain. It's an important symptom.

Visible evidence of arthritis may include ...

- ◆ Swollen joints.

- ◆ Redness and warmth.

- ◆ Tenderness.

- ◆ Diminished strength in muscles around joints.

- ◆ Nodules, which are bumps on or near your joints.

Finally, you can expect your rheumatologist to check the range of motion of the joints that are bothering you. Joints that are swollen, inflamed, and sore won't move as freely and as completely as joints that are functioning normally.

The best time to ask your questions is at the end of the consultation, after the doctor has gathered needed information from your history, your physical, and his review of your previous records and diagnostic studies.

Sometimes all the information you're receiving may seem too much to absorb at one time. Having someone along with you can help a great deal. Have a spouse or friend come along with you to write down the answers as you get them. If you've provided some space after each question on your list, this will be the best place to record it.

Above all, don't feel rushed. If you feel you are being hurried along, say so. Doctors are very busy people, and there are undoubtedly patients in the waiting room waiting for you to leave so they can have their turns. But you are paying for this time. Use it to your best advantage and you'll also reduce the number of follow-up phone calls you make asking for clarifications.

Summing Up

This first rheumatology appointment has covered a great deal of territory, but it may be just the starting point. If you don't receive a definitive diagnosis at this time, don't be surprised and don't be disappointed. The proper diagnosis can take some time. If your primary-care provider hasn't already performed all the needed studies, additional lab tests and X-rays may be needed.

If your rheumatologist is confident that she's made the proper diagnosis during this initial visit, she'll be able to prescribe initial therapy. However, sometimes determining what type of arthritis or other rheumatologic condition you have and prescribing appropriate therapy may require additional testing and follow-up appointments.

Becoming an Active Member of Your Health-Care Team

In many aspects of life it's considered rude to put the focus and spotlight on yourself. When dealing with your health, however, this isn't rude—it's vitally important. No one has more of a vested interest in your health and well-being than you do. Because this is so important, it's critical that you become an informed consumer of health care. Educating yourself about your medical condition will permit you to make the best choices when it comes to getting help.

As your knowledge about arthritis increases, you'll find that your questions have more substance. They'll become more detailed and specific. You'll be learning about what's important for managing your condition. Learning is an ongoing process, and each day more and more information becomes available. Knowledge is empowering, and the more you learn, the more control you will have over the quality of your life.

Precautions

Learn everything you can about your condition, but remember that you aren't a physician (unless you are!) and leave the diagnostics to someone who is trained in that area. Diagnosis involves analyzing symptoms, conducting specific medical tests, and then arriving at sound conclusions.

While it's important to educate yourself about arthritis, you may become confused when faced with all the information that's available on the Internet. Some sites are good and others are not. Ask your rheumatologist for recommendations.

Sometimes too much information can be worse than too little. You may find yourself tailoring your symptoms to conditions that just aren't a good fit. Human nature being what it is, you'll probably choose the worst-case scenario. Read to learn, not to diagnose yourself!

After you receive your diagnosis, your rheumatologist will discuss treatment options with you. These may include either prescription or over-the-counter medications, lifestyle changes, physical or occupational therapy, and perhaps surgery. You'll likely be working with a variety of health-care professionals from this point onward.

Your Medical Team

We live in a time of medical specialization. This has obvious benefits, and it also presents some unique challenges. Today the team approach is commonly used to treat medical conditions, and this works especially well in managing a chronic disease, such as arthritis.

From pain management to therapeutic exercise to surgery, there's a health-care professional trained to provide the best advice and a treatment program designed uniquely for you. Here's a look at the professionals you are likely to work with as you learn to manage and live with arthritis.

Primary-Care Physician

Many milder cases of arthritis are treated perfectly well by primary-care physicians without the need for a referral to a rheumatologist. Even if you are seeing a rheumatologist, your primary-care physician is there to help you and will remain an important member of your health-care team.

Arthritis is one factor in your medical history, but there will be times when your primary-care doctor will be the one you'll call when other illnesses or conditions arise. This physician is the one who referred you to your rheumatologist. In turn, your rheumatologist may refer you to other specialists, as the need arises.

Rheumatologist

The American College of Rheumatology defines a rheumatologist as a physician who treats arthritis, certain immune system diseases, and osteoporosis. After four years of medical school and three years of residency training in internal medicine, rheumatologists devote an additional two to three years in rheumatology-specific training, called a fellowship.

This special training provides expertise in diagnosing and treating the entire gamut of rheumatologic illness, from osteoarthritis to lupus to tennis elbow! Rheumatologists prescribe medications, inject painful joints, and refer patients to therapy, but don't perform surgeries, such as joint replacements.

Physician Assistants

Physician assistants are health-care practitioners authorized to perform diagnostic and therapeutic tasks delegated to them by physicians. Often physician assistants work in rural and other medically underserved areas. They may conduct physical examinations, diagnose medical issues, and prescribe medications. All physician assistants must be associated with a physician. In most states the physician need not be physically present for the physician assistant to practice.

Physician assistants spend an average of 25 months studying an intensive core curriculum that resembles a shortened form of general medical education. To be licensed, physician assistants must pass the national certifying examination of the National Commission on Certification of Physician Assistants, an independent accrediting agency, after which they must complete 100 hours of continuing medical education every two years and pass a recertification examination every six years.

Ophthalmologist

An ophthalmologist is a physician who specializes in treating diseases of the eye. Certain potentially serious complications of some types of arthritis involve the eye. These complications are iritis and uveitis, inflammation of certain portions of the eye. Since these complications can lead to loss of vision, it is important to treat them early. Your rheumatologist will refer you to an ophthalmologist if you develop any eye symptoms.

Orthopedic Surgeon

An orthopedic surgeon, also known as an orthopedist, is a physician who specializes in the diagnosis, treatment, and prevention of problems involving muscles, bones, joints, ligaments, tendons, and nerves.

If you require joint replacement surgery, your physician will refer you to an orthopedic surgeon. Some orthopedic surgeons have subspecialty practices and work only on specific areas of the body, such as the foot, hand, shoulder, spine, hip, or knee. Others may specialize in pediatrics, trauma, or sports medicine.

Advanced Practice Nurses

Advanced practice nurses (APNs) work in collaboration with physicians to provide preventative care and treatment and participate in the management of acute and chronic illnesses, such as arthritis. Nurses are good sources of information and can explain your treatment program in language you can understand.

APNs may be nurse practitioners, clinical nurse specialists, certified nurse midwives, or certified registered nurse anesthetists. Advanced practice nursing is practiced by registered nurses (RNs) who have specialized formal, post-basic education and who function in highly autonomous and specialized roles.

In medical practices that employ them, advanced practice nurses have many functions. Their work may include new patient evaluations prior to seeing the doctor, routine follow-up visits, clinical trials, and processing calls from patients in order of importance.

Occupational and Physical Therapists

When arthritis interferes with your daily life, an occupational therapist can provide you with both assistive devices, such as splints or braces to help support your joints, and information on how to conserve energy while you're performing tasks. There's always an easier way to do things. You'll learn how to make changes in both your home and work settings to reduce strain on your joints.

The occupational therapist will conduct an assessment of your needs and develop a therapy plan designed just for you. Her expertise is solving problems!

A physical therapist will help you regain strength, restore movement, and increase your range of motion in joints that have been affected by arthritis; work to relieve pain; and also help you maintain an optimal fitness level through a program of therapeutic exercise. These health professionals can show you the best way to move from one position to another. They can also teach you how to use walking aids such as crutches, a walker, or a cane when needed.

The physical therapist will also conduct an assessment of your physical strength and range of motion prior to developing your therapy program.

Physical therapy should begin early on to reduce painful symptoms of inflammation, prevent deformity and permanent joint stiffness, and maintain strength in the surrounding muscles.

Mental Health Professionals

You can't separate your mind from your body. Chronic illness can cause symptoms of depression, such as lack of appetite, poor sleep patterns, and feelings of hopelessness.

You may feel at times that you're never going to have a life free from pain. You may fear losing your independence and becoming a burden to your family.

In these difficult times, it can be especially helpful to talk to someone who understands these fears and concerns and who can help you deal with them in a positive manner. Everyone needs help at some time in life.

Consultation

It's not a sign of weakness to admit that you need help coping. It's actually a sign of strength. Getting help is doing something about the problem, and that's good.

There are a variety of specially trained mental health professionals. Psychiatrists, psychologists, and counselors are all available to help you understand the emotional aspects of coping with a chronic illness such as arthritis. Your rheumatologist can refer you.

Podiatrist

When arthritis involves your feet, standing and walking can be quite painful. You may be referred to a podiatrist, a physician who specializes in evaluating and treating diseases of the foot. In addition to prescribing medication or performing surgery, a podiatrist can prescribe special shoes or other devices that can relieve your discomfort.

Dentist

From learning how to brush your teeth when arthritis in your hands makes this chore difficult to finding ways to treat the dry mouth that accompanies Sjögren's syndrome, your dentist is the one to consult for help.

Social Worker

Chronic illness can impact every area of your life. From dealing with financial concerns to changes in the dynamics of family relationships to understanding how insurance companies manage claims, a social worker can help with practical advice, resources, and support.

The Least You Need to Know

- ◆ Symptoms of arthritis can include stiffness, swollen joints, pain, redness, and limited motion in the affected joint.

- ◆ Your rheumatologist is a physician trained to diagnose and treat arthritis and other rheumatologic diseases.

- ◆ Early diagnosis and treatment can prevent many complications associated with arthritis.

- ◆ There is no cure for arthritis, but your health-care team can help you manage your symptoms and lead a productive life.

Part 2

The Different Types of Arthritis

There are more than 100 different kinds of rheumatic conditions, and arthritis itself is a broad term. While these conditions share some similar characteristics, there are also important differences. In Part 2, we'll identify those similarities and differences and gain a clearer understanding of the different forms arthritis can take.

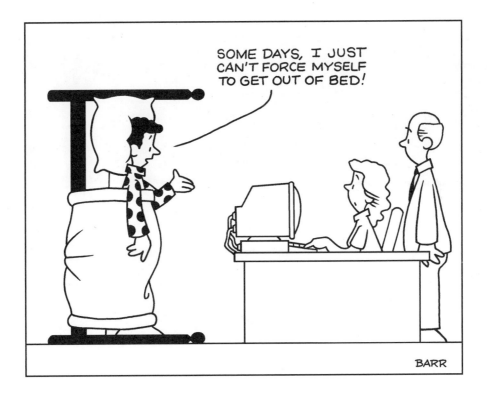

Osteoarthritis

In This Chapter

- ◆ The arthritis of wear and tear
- ◆ Can anyone develop osteoarthritis?
- ◆ Discovering your risk factors
- ◆ Diagnosing osteoarthritis
- ◆ Treatment options

Osteoarthritis (OA) is the most common form of arthritis. It's the one that immediately comes to mind when you think of aching joints. Osteoarthritis affects more than 21 million people in the United States and untold numbers worldwide. Because it's so common, OA can also occur together with other types of arthritis.

What Is Osteoarthritis?

Osteoarthritis is a form of chronic arthritis that attacks the joints—the places where bones meet. In healthy joints, a thin layer of cartilage serves as cushioning material to keep the bones from rubbing together when they move. Cartilage is a protein substance that acts like a shock absorber. It's firm and somewhat rubbery, so it can change shape to accommodate different positions of the joint. It compresses when the joint closes and expands when the joint opens up.

In osteoarthritis, chronic use and low-level inflammation eventually cause the cartilage to lose its elastic properties and become stiff. This leads to thinning and eventual loss of cartilage in some places.

Ligaments become less distensible as we age, more like leather straps than rubber bands. If there is significant loss of cartilage, such as in the knee, the ligaments are then longer than the joints that they cross. That leads to further joint instability and may contribute to pain. The bone overgrows, causing pain, and the joints to appear larger than normal. If the cartilage is damaged severely enough, the ends of the bones meet without that essential cushion, and more pain and damage result.

Consultation

Humans aren't the only species to suffer from osteoarthritis. It appears to affect almost all vertebrates, from porpoises to dinosaurs.

Osteoarthritis usually affects just one joint, although it can target any joint in the body. The hips, the knees, the spine, the hands, and the feet are most often affected. When the hands are afflicted, several finger joints may be involved. Sometimes you'll hear osteoarthritis referred to as *degenerative joint disease*, a term that reflects the inflammation, breakdown, and gradual loss of cartilage in the affected joint.

There are two types of osteoarthritis: primary (the cause is unknown) and secondary (the cause is known). Primary osteoarthritis is generally associated with aging. Secondary osteoarthritis develops as a result of another disease or condition. There are numerous possible causes:

- Obesity
- Repeated trauma to the joint
- Surgical procedures
- Gout
- Pseudogout
- Rheumatoid arthritis
- Diabetes and other hormonal disorders
- Hemochromatosis (a condition that causes iron buildup in the joints)

    ◆ Bleeding disorders (such as hemophilia)

    ◆ Congenital joint defects

In addition to the breakdown of cartilage in osteoarthritis, the bones themselves can undergo changes, enlarging and forming bone spurs called osteophytes. The joint lining (synovium) and joint capsule can also undergo changes that result in loss of movement and pain. Different joints are affected differently.

Who Gets Osteoarthritis?

Just about anyone can develop OA. Osteoarthritis occurs across the population. It does not discriminate on the basis of race, gender, or even age. Younger people and athletes can develop osteoarthritis after injuring a joint. Generally, though, OA tends to occur with greater frequency as we (and our joints) age. Men are more susceptible to osteoarthritis before the age of 45, but women take the lead after age 55.

Researchers believe that a genetic component of OA is responsible for these differences, and that joint angles or other elements of body structure particular to specific racial groups may play a role.

What Causes Osteoarthritis?

That's a direct, simple question without a direct, simple answer. Researchers do not yet know what's behind the initial breakdown of cartilage that eventually develops into OA. What they do know, however, is that certain risk factors can increase your chances of developing osteoarthritis. If you have a combination of risk factors, your potential for OA increases.

Obesity

If there is one risk factor you have some control over, this is it. Why is weight important? Excess weight puts extra stress on your weight-bearing joints, including your hips and knees. Losing as little as 10 pounds can significantly reduce your chances of developing osteoarthritis in your knees. If you already have knee OA, losing weight can help you feel better.

So what is obesity? You used to be able to glance at a chart that gave a list of heights and appropriate weight ranges. All that changed, however, when scientists determined these were not accurate measures of overall health.

def•i•ni•tion

Body mass index (BMI) relates your weight to your height. Your BMI is your weight in kilograms (kg) divided by your height in meters (m) squared. This figure correlates strongly with total body fat content in adults.

The National Institutes of Health (NIH) has turned instead to the *body mass index* (BMI) to define normal weight, overweight, and obesity. For women, a BMI of 27.3 or above is considered overweight; for men, 27.8 or above. A BMI of 30 or above is considered obese.

Quite a bit of research has been done to discover how obesity and osteoarthritis are related. One study found a hormonal connection: a hormone called leptin that is associated with obesity is also found in higher levels in people with knee OA.

A British study found a strong connection between obesity and OA. The researchers determined that the risk of knee OA increased 40 percent for each 10 pounds of weight a woman gained. They concluded that if obese individuals reduced their weights to fall within the normal range, 24 percent of surgeries for knee OA might be avoided. The results were published in the *International Journal of Obesity* (2001).

To put this research into simple terms, each pound you weigh puts at least three pounds of stress on your knees and even more on your hips. This continued stress can eventually alter the normal joint structure. Losing 5 pounds reduces the stress load by 15 pounds for your knees. That's a significant load lifter!

def•i•ni•tion

Longitudinal studies follow the same people over an extended period of time. They are important in understanding how disease develops and how successful medications are in treating disease.

Obesity has also been linked to an increased risk of hand OA. The Tecumseh Community Health Study in Michigan was a *longitudinal study* that looked at the role of obesity in the development of osteoarthritis.

The study, which ran from 1962 to 1985, involved about 1,200 men and women. At the end of the study, the ages of the participants ranged from 50 to 74 years. Researchers found that the more obese an individual was at the beginning of the study, the greater the subsequent severity of hand OA. This was true even for those who didn't have hand OA at the beginning of the study, but who developed it later on.

Heredity

Your genes definitely play a role in whether or not you will develop osteoarthritis. If you were born with abnormalities of certain joints or cartilage defects, daily wear and tear will eventually take its toll, causing earlier cartilage breakdown. If your joints don't meet correctly, if one leg is shorter than the other, or if you are pigeon-toed, outward-toed, knock-kneed (knees angle inward), or bow-legged (knees angle out), your walking patterns put stress on your joints, and over time, you are more likely to develop osteoarthritis in those joints. Genetics is believed to be involved in about half of hand and hip OA cases and a slightly lower percentage of knee OA cases.

Identifying the particular gene or genes responsible for OA takes time, money, persistence, and more than a little luck. Sometimes the findings come in interesting ways. For example, researchers have discovered a connection between shortness and increased risk for osteoarthritis. Having shorter bones and less cartilage may make joints more susceptible to damage. But the opposite condition may also contribute to OA: taller people's longer bones may increase stress on the joints. Since many genes control height, but only a few genes are associated with arthritis, this research has narrowed the possibilities for the genes responsible for OA. The study was reported in the journal *Nature Genetics* (January 2008). Other studies have reinforced the genetic connection:

- In a study comparing identical and non-identical twins, researchers found that if one identical twin had OA, the other twin was twice as likely to also develop OA of the hand or knee.

- Sisters of women who had hand OA were found to be twice as likely as the general population to develop hand OA. The risk jumped five to seven times if the sister had a severe case.

- Certain gene mutations have been linked to specific OA sites, such as the hand, hip, or knee. This may mean that each joint has an individual genetic basis for developing OA.

Osteoarthritis may primarily be associated with aging, but we are learning that genetics may set the stage before we're even born.

Aging

As we age, so do the joints in our body. Osteoarthritis has traditionally been associated with aging, and its occurrence definitely increases with age. It's the most commonly reported chronic medical condition in those over the age of 65, with more than 80 percent of those age 75 and over affected. It is uncommon in those under age 40.

The greatest increase in osteoarthritis is occurring in individuals between the ages of 40 and 50. As the Boomer generation ages, their numbers will have a definite influence on osteoarthritis statistics. According to estimates by the National Arthritis Data Workgroup, about one third of Americans aged 25 to 74 have osteoarthritis as determined by X-rays of the hand, foot, knee, or hip joints. However, only about half of these people will ever develop symptoms.

Gender

Generally, women are more prone to develop osteoarthritis than men. After age 55, women have a higher occurrence of OA of the knee than do men. Some research indicates that menopause and decreased production of estrogen may play a role here, since estrogen replacement therapy has been linked with a decreased risk of developing OA.

Other studies have found that women have more involvement of multiple joints and greater and more severe OA of the hands, knees, ankles, and feet. Men, however, seem to have a greater occurrence and severity of OA of the hips, wrist, and spine.

Men are more prone to develop osteoarthritis under age 45 than are women, usually involving one or two joints. After age 44, rates of OA increase more rapidly for women. After age 55, OA occurs more often in women and tends to involve multiple joints. The Tecumseh study mentioned earlier found that hand and wrist OA affected 78 percent of the men and 90 percent of the women aged 65 and above.

Joint Injury and Joint Overuse

Sports injuries, accidents, and repeated minor trauma to joints and cartilage can all contribute to the development of osteoarthritis. So can repetitive motions that put stress on your weight-bearing joints, such as kneeling or squatting. OA develops more rapidly in older adults who have sustained previous joint injuries.

Precautions

Treat injuries to your joints early on to prevent possible development of OA later on. Have torn ligaments repaired and take advantage of physical therapy to safeguard your joints.

Your occupation may also determine whether or not you develop OA. An English study reported in *Annals of the Rheumatic Diseases* (2006) focused on coal miners found that frequent or prolonged kneeling or squatting (positions associated with mining) doubled their risk of developing knee OA. Heavy lifting increased that risk still more. A French study found that cleaning women and women employed in the clothing industry suffered from osteoarthritis at rates five to six times that of the general population and had a unique pattern of hip, knee, and hand involvement. The repetitive motions involved in these occupations were blamed. Among construction workers, both men and women were found to have three times the occurrence of hip and knee OA of those not in the field. These studies were reported in the *American Journal of Epidemiology* (1998).

Other risk factors include ...

- ◆ **Joint infection.** On rare occasions, bacteria, viruses, and fungi can enter a joint. They cause damage and set the stage for the development of osteoarthritis. Among these troublesome invaders are the bacteria that cause Lyme disease and gonorrhea.

- ◆ **Muscle weakness.** In individuals over age 65, osteoarthritis of the knee has been associated with weakness in the quadriceps, the muscle that extends from the front of the thigh across the knee and down the shin. As we age, muscle weakness causes the knee to lose some of its stability, which seems to increase the potential for developing osteoarthritis.

Any kind of repetitive motion can wear away at the joint over time and eventually lead to OA. Many factors are involved in the development of OA, and researchers are studying how they work.

But there's always the exception to the rule! Marathon runners have a relatively low occurrence of OA. It may be that running leads to healthy cartilage. The rhythmic compression of cartilage that occurs during running may expel wastes and encourage the absorption of nutrients. This may also be a matter of self-selection. Runners who develop joint pain are likely to change to biking or walking. In addition, most marathoners are quite slender.

Arriving at a Diagnosis

No single test can determine if you have osteoarthritis. A diagnosis of OA is based on a combination of factors, including your description of symptoms, the location and pattern of the pain, and the results of a physical examination, which may include tests and screenings such as X-rays or an MRI. Unlike in rheumatoid arthritis, which we'll discuss in Chapter 4, there are no blood test abnormalities associated with OA.

Your physician will look at X-rays to see if you have loss of cartilage. If the space between the bones in the joint is narrower than it should be, if bone density near the joint has increased beyond normal levels, or if bony growths or cysts are present—all these are indicators for osteoarthritis.

Signs and Symptoms

The symptoms of osteoarthritis often develop gradually over many years and can come and go. Some individuals with significant joint deterioration may experience few symptoms, while others with similar levels of deterioration may be disabled by their symptoms.

Consultation

Reading an X-ray takes a trained eye. Bones are dense and appear white on an X-ray. Air is black, and other structures appear as different shades of gray, depending on their density.

Pain is the most common symptom, worsening with activity and improving after rest. This means that you experience more pain as the day goes on. However, you may also experience pain after periods of inactivity. The pain, often described as aching, can be worse in humid weather. Stiffness and loss of mobility in the affected joint accompany the pain. If your knee is involved, you may hear a crackling sound (crepitus) when you move it. (This is probably the origin of the phrase "old and decrepit.")

If you have swelling or stiffness in your joints lasting more than two weeks, it's time to make an appointment to see your physician.

Medical Tests and Screenings

During your physical examination, your doctor will look for tender areas, redness, warmth, stiffness, reduced range of motion, and fluid in your joints. Your doctor will ask about your and your family's medical histories and may perform blood tests, urine tests, X-rays and other imaging tests, and joint aspiration (removal of fluid from the affected joint).

Enlarged joints may be caused by the formation of bone spurs, called Heberden's nodes, Bouchard's nodes, or bunions. Heberden's nodes are pea-sized or smaller knots found on the first finger joints below the fingertips. Bouchard's nodes are found on the middle finger joint. Bunions form at the joints at the base of the big toes. If bone spurs are present, they can aid in the diagnosis of osteoarthritis.

There is no blood test that can diagnose osteoarthritis. A blood test is used to rule out certain diseases that can cause secondary arthritis or other arthritic conditions.

X-rays can reveal how much joint damage has taken place. They can show any narrowing of the space between the bones in the joint (a result of cartilage loss) and whether bone spurs have formed. X-rays are also helpful in determining whether surgery may be helpful.

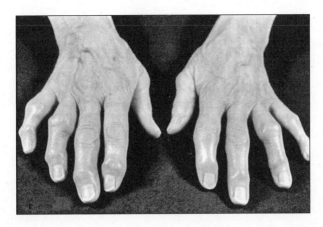

Osteoarthritis: Heberden's &
Bouchard's Nodes.

Photo courtesy of the American
College of Rheumatology

If fluid has accumulated in a joint, your physician can use a sterile needle to withdraw some of it for analysis, a procedure called joint aspiration or arthrocentesis (see Chapter 10). This analysis can rule out certain secondary arthritic conditions, including gout and infection.

Treatment

There are many treatment options for osteoarthritis, and your treatment will depend in large extent on the severity of your symptoms. Milder symptoms will generally be treated with lifestyle changes, physical and occupational therapy, and some medications. Recommendations for important lifestyle changes include …

- Losing excess weight.

- Committing to a program of regular low-impact exercise.

- Resting sore joints to decrease stress, pain, and swelling.

- Reducing the intensity and duration of activities that cause joint pain.

- Listening to what your body is telling you.

- Asking for help when you need it. Don't try to be superman or super-woman.

Consultation

A weight-loss program combined with an exercise program has been proven to produce more effective pain relief and greater joint function than either weight loss or exercise alone.

If your work requires repetitive motions that stress your joints, you'll want to look into ways to perform your job without putting extra strain on your joints. In some cases this may mean transferring jobs within a company or even switching to a line of work that doesn't cause your symptoms to worsen.

For more severe cases of osteoarthritis, your rheumatologist has additional options, including stronger medications and a referral to an orthopedic surgeon.

Medications

A wide variety of medications, both prescription and over-the-counter, is available to treat the pain and inflammation of osteoarthritis. For complete arthritis drug information, including side effects, see Chapter 9.

To start, your rheumatologist may prescribe pain-relieving medications, such as acetaminophen (Tylenol). Acetaminophen has fewer gastrointestinal side effects than aspirin, ibuprofen, or naproxen, which are used to treat both pain and inflammation.

Topical treatments, such as creams and ointments, applied to the skin over the painful area may be beneficial. These topicals include capsaicin (ArthriCare, Zostrix), salycin (Aspercreme), methyl salicylate (Bengay, Icy Hot), and menthol (Flexall). Additionally, ice packs can provide soothing relief.

If oral and topical medications don't provide you relief, injections of steroids directly into the affected joint may be an option. For this procedure, your physician will numb the area around the joint, insert a sterile needle into the joint space, and inject the medication. More than two, or at most three, steroid injections per year into any one joint are not recommended. Overusing steroid injections can lead to the breakdown of cartilage and bone.

If you suffer from knee OA and other medications have not relieved your pain, your rheumatologist or orthopedic surgeon may recommend injections of hyaluronic acid derivatives into your knee joint. This procedure, known as viscosupplementation, has been approved by the FDA to treat the pain of knee OA. Several preparations of hyaluronic acid are now commercially available. These medications include Synvisc, Supartz, Euflexxa, Orthovisc, and Hyalgan. Depending upon which medication your physician uses, you will receive three to five injections over a period of several weeks.

Hyaluronic acid occurs naturally in the joint fluid and acts as a lubricant and cushion for the knee joint. It may also have anti-inflammatory and pain-relieving properties. In knee OA, natural levels of hyaluronic acid are lower than normal. Injections of hyaluronic acid relieve pain and may stimulate the body to produce more of its own hyaluronic acid.

After the injection, you may experience some pain, swelling, and warmth at the site. These symptoms are generally short-lived, and ice packs help ease the discomfort. You'll be instructed to avoid excessive standing, heavy lifting, or jogging for the first 48 hours following the injection.

The benefits of these injections, while not immediate, may last for several months, although a significant number of people are not helped by them. Viscosupplementation is also quite expensive. Check with your insurance carrier to see if this treatment is covered under your policy.

Precautions

The material injected in viscosupplementation therapy is derived from purified rooster combs. If you are allergic to birds, feathers, or eggs, you should not have this therapy.

Physical Therapy

Physical therapy has two goals: to decrease pain and to increase the range of motion for your joints. Limited range of motion has a negative impact on most of your daily activities, and the less you use the affected joint, the weaker it will become.

Strengthening the muscles around your joint will help stabilize it. To accomplish this, your physical therapist will use a combination of range-of-motion and strengthening exercises, along with heat and cold therapy. You'll read more about physical therapy in Chapter 17.

Applying heat to the affected joint before you begin therapy increases blood flow to that joint. After therapy, cold packs can be used to reduce inflammation.

A study conducted at Brooke Army Medical Center in Fort Sam Houston, Texas, confirmed the beneficial effects of physical therapy on osteoarthritis. The study found that patients with knee OA who were treated with manual physical therapy and exercise experienced measurably significant improvements in their pain, stiffness, and ability to use their knee. One year later, the benefits remained and the treatment group had undergone fewer knee replacement surgeries.

Exercise

Low-impact activities that don't jar your joints are best; this means saying no to rac-quetball and yes to swimming. Rather than feeling limited by osteoarthritis, consider trying new activities. Walking is still the best bet, and cycling is good as well. You're aiming to strengthen your joints by keeping them moving.

If you're exercising properly, you usually won't aggra-vate osteoarthritis and will help keep your joints from freezing up. You're working to strengthen the muscles that support your joints, as well.

Being even a little overweight puts added stress on your joints, and exercise will help you manage that weight and increase your stamina.

> **Straight Talk**
>
> Motion is lotion. Keep your joints moving to prevent stiffness.
>
> —Ryan York, physical therapist for Pro-Active Physical Therapy

The Arthritis Foundation sponsors exercise programs throughout the United States. Go to www.arthritis.org to see what's available in your area. Your local hospital is also a good place to look for resources.

Surgery

When medication and lifestyle changes don't help, the pain is unrelenting, and stiff-ness prevents you from using your joints, it may be time to consider surgery. There are several different kinds of surgery for osteoarthritis:

- Removing damaged cartilage (arthroscopy)
- Joint replacement (arthroplasty)
- Creating a false joint with scar tissue (resection arthroplasty)
- Realigning bones (osteotomy)
- Fusing joints (arthrodesis)

You'll read about each of these procedures in detail in Chapter 10.

Prognosis Concerns

Osteoarthritis is a chronic, progressive disease. As of now, there is no cure, and treatment and prognosis largely depend upon each individual's response to lifestyle changes, medication, surgery, and other available therapies.

New treatments to block the enzyme responsible for damaging and destroying cartilage tissue or to block the processes that create these enzymes are currently under development. Also on the horizon are therapies designed to stimulate the production of new joint tissue or replace the damaged tissue.

The Least You Need to Know

- ◆ Osteoarthritis is the most common type of arthritis.
- ◆ Maintaining a healthy weight is key to preventing osteoarthritis.
- ◆ Injuries to your joints can cause osteoarthritis later in life.
- ◆ Your occupation may play a role in whether you develop osteoarthritis.
- ◆ Lifestyle changes and medication are the first treatments recommended for osteoarthritis.
- ◆ If lifestyle changes and medications fail, surgery is an option.

Chapter 4

Rheumatoid Arthritis

In This Chapter

◆ The most common form of inflammatory arthritis

◆ Who is affected by rheumatoid arthritis?

◆ Causes and risk factors

◆ Recognizing the signs and symptoms

◆ Diagnosing and treating rheumatoid arthritis

◆ A promising future

Rheumatoid arthritis (RA) is an autoimmune disease that causes chronic joint inflammation and swelling. RA can vary widely in symptoms and outcomes and is the arthritic condition most associated with joint deformity and disability. Today there are new treatments available for this serious form of arthritis, and the outlook is improving.

What Is Rheumatoid Arthritis?

Rheumatoid arthritis is the most common form of inflammatory arthritis. It attacks the joint lining, called the synovium, causing swelling and pain. Eventually, RA damages the joint itself. The pain and swelling of RA can make even routine tasks extremely difficult. This is the type of arthritis that brings to mind pictures of swollen and deformed joints, especially of the hands.

Rheumatoid arthritis develops in two stages. The first stage involves swelling of the joint lining. This causes the symptoms of pain, stiffness, redness, swelling, and warmth around the joint. In the second stage, the inflamed cells release certain enzymes. These enzymes actually digest the bone and cartilage, which makes the joint lose both its shape and its alignment. More pain and loss of movement then occur.

Early treatment of your rheumatoid arthritis will make you feel better, more likely to be able to lead an active life, and less likely to experience the type of joint damage that leads to joint replacement.

Who Gets Rheumatoid Arthritis?

RA affects 1.3 million Americans. Generally, it tends to occur most often between the ages of 40 and 60, although children can also develop RA. About 75 percent of individuals who have rheumatoid arthritis are women, although its symptoms tend to be more severe in men.

There is likely a genetic component to rheumatoid arthritis. Studies of identical twins have found that if one twin develops RA, the other twin is much more likely than a non-identical twin or another sibling to also develop RA.

Precautions

Rheumatoid arthritis may go into remission in pregnant women, although symptoms tend to flare after the baby's birth. RA also develops more often than expected in the year after giving birth. Researchers are studying the effects female hormones might have on the development of RA.

Causes and Risk Factors for Rheumatoid Arthritis

The exact cause of rheumatoid arthritis is not yet known, but it appears that a combination of factors is responsible. We do know that rheumatoid arthritis is an autoimmune disease. This means that it develops when something goes wrong with your body's immune system, the system that's supposed to protect you from infection. In an autoimmune disease, the body turns on itself and attacks its own tissues. Why this happens is being studied.

Certain genetic markers, including a marker called human lymphocyte antigen (HLA-DR4), are more common among people who have rheumatoid arthritis than among people who don't. Having this marker doesn't mean that you have or will develop RA. It just means that you are at increased risk. Researchers have also identified other genes that seem to influence the development and the severity of RA. The presence of an abnormal gene may increase the risk of activating the body's immune response when there's an environmental trigger, such as smoking, or exposure to an infectious agent, such as a virus, bacteria, or fungus.

A study reported in the September 6, 2007, issue of the *New England Journal of Medicine* identified a genetic risk factor for both rheumatoid arthritis and lupus. The gene, STAT4, encodes a protein that plays an important role in the regulation and activation of certain cells of the immune system. Identifying the genes responsible is the first step toward a cure.

It's possible that you may inherit a predisposition to developing RA. If you have a family member with rheumatoid arthritis, you have an increased chance of developing RA.

Precautions

Smoking cigarettes has been found to increase your risk of developing rheumatoid arthritis. The reason why isn't yet known, but to reduce your chances of developing RA, quitting smoking is one of the best decisions you can make.

Immune System Malfunction

In a healthy immune system, white blood cells produce antibodies that protect the body against viruses and bacterial infections. However, when the white blood cells responsible for fighting off infection travel away from the bloodstream and move into a joint lining, they cause trouble rather than fight it. It appears that they play a part in causing the joint lining to become inflamed.

Inflammation causes the release of certain proteins that, over time, cause the joint lining to thicken. The proteins also damage the cartilage, bone, tendons, and ligaments around the joint. This leads to swelling and eventually to cartilage and bone damage. The joint eventually loses its shape and alignment, and it may even be destroyed.

The Role of Rheumatoid Factor

Rheumatoid factor (RF) is an *antibody* that can bind to other antibodies. These antibodies are normal proteins found in the blood and are part of the immune system. Rheumatoid factor is found in about 1–2 percent of healthy people, and its prevalence increases with age. About 20 percent of people age 65 and older have an elevated rheumatoid factor.

def•i•ni•tion

An **antibody** is a type of protein made by certain white blood cells in response to the presence of a foreign substance, called an antigen.

If you have a high rheumatoid factor level, your immune system might be malfunctioning. Your doctor will often order a blood test to measure rheumatoid factor to help arrive at a diagnosis of rheumatoid arthritis.

Not everyone with RA has an elevated rheumatoid factor and not everyone with an elevated rheumatoid factor has RA. Generally, though, the higher the level of rheumatoid factor present in the body, the more severe the disease activity is.

Infection

Some researchers and physicians think that a bacterial or viral infection can trigger an autoimmune response that may lead to rheumatoid arthritis. This is being researched, and currently there is no proof that this is true. It may be that some people who carry a genetic susceptibility to RA have immune systems that react differently to infectious agents than people without this genetic inclination.

Signs and Symptoms

The signs and symptoms of rheumatoid arthritis can include joint pain, swelling, and tenderness. Rheumatoid arthritis most commonly begins in the smaller joints of the fingers, hands, and wrists, and the pattern is usually symmetrical, meaning that if a joint hurts on your left hand, the same joint will hurt on your right hand. The following illustration shows how rheumatoid arthritis affects the fingers.

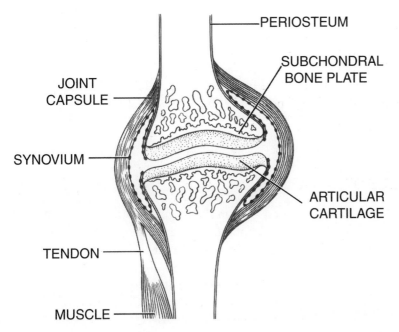

PERIOSTEUM

SUBCHONDRAL
BONE PLATE

JOINT
CAPSULE

SYNOVIUM

ARTICULAR
CARTILAGE

TENDON

MUSCLE

Soft tissue swelling (synovitis) of the PIP joints in rheumatoid arthritis.

In addition, you may notice that your hands are red and puffy and there are firm bumps, called rheumatoid nodules, under the skin on your hands and arms. Other symptoms can include …

♦ Fatigue.

♦ Morning stiffness that lasts at least 30 minutes.

♦ Low-grade fever.

♦ Loss of appetite and weight loss.

♦ Decreased energy level.

♦ Dry eyes and mouth from an associated condition known as Sjögren's syndrome (see Chapter 8).

The symptoms of RA can come and go. There may be periods when symptoms lessen or even go away. These periods are followed by periods of increased disease activity known as flares.

Rheumatoid arthritis is a systemic disease. This means that it can affect other organs in the body in addition to involving the joints. Lung tissues can become inflamed, which can cause chest pain when you cough or breathe deeply. Sometimes rheumatoid nodules develop in the lungs.

If the tissue surrounding your heart becomes inflamed, a condition known as pericarditis, you may have chest pain that changes in intensity with different body movements, such as lying down or leaning forward.

While other types of arthritis may cause stiffness first thing in the morning or after periods of inactivity, the kind of stiffness associated with RA is longer lasting. It's usually at its worst in the morning and generally lasts from one to two hours, although it may last all day long.

Arriving at a Diagnosis

A complete physical examination is the first step on the journey toward an accurate diagnosis. Your physician will ask you what symptoms you are experiencing and take your complete medical history. As you read in Chapter 2, it's important that you come to your appointment prepared to answer your doctor's questions (and with questions of your own). What kinds of questions are you likely to be asked?

- Do you feel stiff in the morning?

- How long does the stiffness last?

- Have you been feeling fatigued during the day?

- Are your joints painful? Which ones?

- Does the same joint hurt on both sides of your body or does it just hurt on one side?

- Do you have joint pain in many joints?

- When is the pain most severe?

Consultation

Self-report scales are also used to give your rheumatologist information on how you're doing. Two of the most common are the Health Assessment Questionnaire (HAQ) and the Arthritis Impact Measurement Scales (AIMS).

You can expect to answer these questions each time you visit the doctor. This helps him see how you're doing and whether your medications are effective or if changes need to be made.

After the question and answer session, your doctor will conduct a thorough physical examination. He'll be looking for evidence of joint swelling and tenderness. He'll check to see if your joints are out of alignment and determine if your range of motion in those joints has decreased. He'll also look for signs of rheumatoid arthritis in other parts of the body, including your skin, lungs, and eyes. After the examination is completed, he may order other diagnostic tests and screenings to assist in making a diagnosis.

Blood Work

A considerable amount of data can be gathered from the blood sample taken in the doctor's office and sent to a medical laboratory for analysis. For example, if your red blood cell count is low, you may be anemic. Anemia is common among people who have rheumatoid arthritis. Extreme fatigue can be a symptom of anemia. The more severe your RA, the more anemic you may be.

You may notice the term *complete blood count (CBC)* on your lab report. This means that your red blood cells, white blood cells, and platelets (which help your blood clot) have been tested to check for abnormalities, to monitor side effects of drugs, or to check your progress.

Your rheumatologist will be checking the erythrocyte sedimentation rate, also referred to as *ESR* or *sed rate*. This is a blood test that detects inflammation by measuring how fast red blood cells fall to the bottom of a test tube. The faster they drop out of suspension (the higher the sed rate), the more inflammation is present in your body and the more severe your RA is. This sed rate will be checked frequently to see how well your medications are performing.

When inflammation is present, it also causes levels of a certain protein (C-reactive protein, referred to as *CRP*) to increase. High levels of CRP correspond to higher levels of disease activity. To complicate matters, the sed rate and the CRP don't always work in sync. One may be elevated while the other isn't. Still, CRP is one more test to discover how your RA is progressing. This test may be repeated regularly to monitor your inflammation and your response to medication.

Your blood work will also reveal if you have rheumatoid factor (discussed earlier in the chapter).

Anti-CCP antibody is a fairly recent test for rheumatoid arthritis. It's sometimes positive earlier in the course of the arthritis than rheumatoid factor and is more specific (fewer false positives) for RA. For instance, patients with hepatitis C are frequently RF positive but should be anti-CCP negative.

Finally, your blood work will show if you have antinuclear antibodies (ANA).

Other Tests and Screenings

In addition to blood work, your rheumatologist has other means of assessing your symptoms. Your rheumatologist may draw some fluid from one of your affected joints and send it to the medical laboratory for analysis. This process, called joint fluid aspiration or arthrocentesis, is discussed in Chapter 10. You may notice some relief from your pain after this procedure, as draining some of the fluid can relieve pressure within the joint.

X-rays are generally taken at this first rheumatology appointment. They're helpful as a diagnostic tool, but they may not show many changes in the first three to six months of the course of RA. They're used to establish a baseline. Later on, they may show the presence of bony erosions in the joints, a typical feature of RA. The following illustration shows how these erosions develop over time.

Serial X-rays of a finger in a patient with rheumatoid arthritis showing progressive joint damage (erosions) over time.

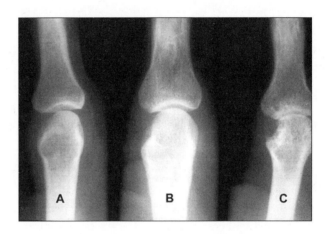

Consultation

X-rays have been used as a diagnostic tool for over 100 years. They were discovered by Wilhelm Röntgen in 1895, and the first X-ray taken was of his wife's hand. He received the first Nobel Prize in Physics in 1901 for his revolutionary discovery.

Newer technology today gives us even clearer images than X-rays. Magnetic resonance imaging (MRI) can detect early inflammation of a joint lining before it is visible on an X-ray. The earlier your physician can detect inflammation, the earlier you can begin your treatment program and reduce the chances of long-term disability and joint deformity.

A screening your rheumatologist may recommend later on is a bone density screening. Known as DEXA, this scan is used primarily to detect osteoporosis, which can be a complication of rheumatoid arthritis or its treatment. A tendency to be inactive because of pain, inflammation itself, and the long-term effects of certain medications, such as steroids, may speed up the process of bone loss. It's important to keep tabs on this.

Ultimately, there is no one specific test that will tell you and your rheumatologist if you have rheumatoid arthritis. Arriving at a diagnosis involves analyzing all the information gathered from your medical history, symptoms, and the tests and screenings that are done, and ruling out the possibility of other diseases.

Treatment

Once your diagnosis has been made, it's time to consider your options for treatment. It's likely to be a full-spectrum approach, including medications, exercise blended with rest, and joint protection. You'll also learn many strategies for managing RA. Many new treatments have been developed over the last 10 years, a result of research into the fundamentals of inflammation. New medications block certain signals from the immune system that result in the symptoms of rheumatoid arthritis and cause joint damage.

Your treatment plan will be tailored to your own symptoms and stage of rheumatoid arthritis, but most likely you'll begin with specific medications designed to reduce inflammation, relieve your pain, stop or slow joint damage, and improve your ability to live life fully.

Remember that it may take a little time to find the best medication and the best dosage to treat your symptoms. Your rheumatologist will most likely start with one of the nonsteroidal anti-inflammatory drugs (NSAIDs). Many of these are now available over the counter without a prescription. They include ibuprofen (Motrin, Advil), naproxen (Aleve, Naprosyn), and celecoxib (Celebrex). In addition to these NSAIDs, your rheumatologist may prescribe low dosages of corticosteroids, such as prednisone.

In addition to NSAIDS and/or low-dose steroids, patients with RA should be on one or more drugs called disease-modifying antirheumatic drugs (DMARDs). These are often used in conjunction with NSAIDs or low-dose corticosteroids. DMARDs have been shown to be quite effective not just in managing symptoms, but also have been proven in scientific studies to slow or halt the rate of damage to joints as measured by serial X-rays. The most commonly used DMARD for treating RA is methotrexate. For more information on DMARDS, see Chapter 9.

If these medications aren't effective for you, there are still more options. One of the most exciting developments in treating rheumatoid arthritis is the arrival of the class of drugs known as biologic response modifiers (*biologics* for short). These have the ability to target specific parts of the immune system that cause inflammation. These drugs directly modify the immune system by inhibiting proteins called cytokines, or lymphocytes, cells that play a major role in the immune process, which contribute to inflammation. They also home in on areas where joint and tissue damage is occurring and actually can slow the progression of this damage.

The biologics may be used by themselves or they may be used in combination with methotrexate to boost their effectiveness. Biologics are discussed in Chapter 9.

If medications aren't enough to stop or slow the progression of joint damage, it may be time to consider surgery to replace or repair the damaged joints. Joint replacement surgery can be quite successful in restoring function and relieving the pain associated with rheumatoid arthritis. Especially when damage has caused deformity of the joint, a replacement can make a world of difference in your ability to function and your general sense of well-being. Surgeries for rheumatoid arthritis include …

- Total joint replacement (arthroplasty).

- Tendon repair.

- Removal of the joint lining (synovectomy), usually performed by arthroscopy.

- Joint fusion (arthrodesis).

All surgeries have certain risks and possible complications, so it's important to educate yourself about the procedures you are considering. You'll find more detailed information on surgeries for arthritis in Chapter 10.

Physical therapy (PT) can help you strengthen your joints and the muscles that surround them. You may find that exercise is painful, but it's important to keep your joints moving. Your physical therapist will work with you to develop a program of therapeutic exercise that you'll be able to follow at home.

When your disease is active and you're going through a flare, listen to your body. This is the time when rest is important. When fatigue, inflammation, and pain make movement difficult, it's time to slow down your exercise program. Gentle range-of-motion exercise will keep your joints flexible and won't put undue strain on them. Walking may be the best kind of exercise you can do. For more on exercising with arthritis, see Chapter 17.

Rheumatoid Arthritis and the Workplace

When rheumatoid arthritis results in disability, it can cause you problems at work. Researchers estimate that up to 39 percent of individuals with early RA leave the workforce within five years of being diagnosed. A 2007 study that appeared in the journal *Arthritis and Rheumatism* found that, despite a decrease in disease activity, the rate at which women with rheumatoid arthritis left the workforce didn't fall significantly between 1987 and 1998.

The 1987 cohort consisted of 48 women, and the 1998 cohort held 91 women. In both groups, more than 25 percent of the women stopped working within four years of being diagnosed with rheumatoid arthritis. Most of the participants were Caucasian, married, and over the age of 50. Researchers were surprised at the results but speculated that other factors may have influenced the women's decisions.

Another study examined risk factors for rheumatoid arthritis–related work disability, which the researchers defined as unemployment, in 469 adults with RA. They found that commuting difficulties, physically demanding jobs, greater joint pain with poor functionality, and nonprofessional or nonadministrative jobs were important predictors of job loss. Those individuals with professional positions fared better.

> **Straight Talk**
>
> I had to have my husband drive me to work. RA made me so tired I couldn't have handled both the drive and the job. It was one or the other.
>
> —Celeste, age 45

There are strategies available to help you remain employed and more comfortable at work. See Chapter 19 for a discussion of those strategies.

Prognosis Concerns

Research is ongoing into the causes and a cure for RA. One exciting area is gene therapy, and this research is moving in some interesting directions. In the future …

◆ Specific genes in your body may be programmed to direct cells to manufacture substances that would reduce inflammation.

◆ You may receive a new healthy gene to replace a gene that is defective.

◆ It may be possible to turn off a harmful gene.

Very small studies involving humans have been conducted and have shown some promise. Gene therapy is still many years away from being used to treat arthritis, but the work is continuing.

The prognosis for living with rheumatoid arthritis is much brighter today than at any time in the past. New treatments, especially the biologic medications, have proven to have a remarkable effect on the course of this disease.

The National Institutes of Health (NIH) sponsors clinical trials for new treatments for RA. If you are interested in participating, go to the website clinicaltrials.gov for more information. Many rheumatologists, both in private practice and at medical schools, also participate in clinical trials of promising new drugs for those RA patients not adequately controlled by those agents already on the market.

Early diagnosis and treatment still provide the best chances of minimizing the disabling effects of rheumatoid arthritis, and it's critical to seek medical advice early. The risk of heart disease and stroke is higher for people with RA, so it's important for your overall health and well-being to keep in close contact with your rheumatologist.

You can continue to lead a full and productive life while dealing with rheumatoid arthritis. The key is in seeking the best medical advice, following through with your treatment and therapy programs, and keeping a positive attitude.

The Least You Need to Know

- Rheumatoid arthritis is an autoimmune disease that causes chronic inflammation involving joints and other organs.

- Women are at greater risk for RA than men.

- If medications aren't enough to stop or slow down the progression of joint damage, joint replacement surgery may be necessary.

- Treating RA early can help prevent joint deformity and slow the progression of the disease.

- New treatments, such as the biologics, have dramatically improved the prognosis for people with RA.

Juvenile Arthritis

In This Chapter

- ◆ Young people and arthritis
- ◆ Factors that may cause juvenile arthritis
- ◆ What are the symptoms?
- ◆ Diagnosis and treatment options
- ◆ Putting together your child's medical team
- ◆ Prognosis and remission

Juvenile arthritis (JA) is the most common form of arthritis affecting children. Current estimates put the number of children in the United States with JA at over 300,000. Juvenile arthritis was formerly called juvenile rheumatoid arthritis, but the name was changed to more accurately reflect the diverse forms of the condition. Health-care professionals prefer to call it juvenile idiopathic arthritis (JIA), a term indicating that the cause or causes of juvenile arthritis are not yet known. Recognizing the signs and symptoms of juvenile arthritis, arriving at a diagnosis, and developing a treatment plan are key to managing JA.

What Is Juvenile Arthritis?

Juvenile arthritis is a type of arthritis that affects children under the age of 16. It is a chronic condition that may also affect other organs in the body. As with other forms of arthritis, pain, fatigue, and joint inflammation are among its main symptoms.

There are three main kinds of juvenile arthritis. Two of them have names that reflect the number of joints affected by JA. The third kind affects the child's organs in addition to the joints.

Juvenile Arthritis (One to Four Joints)

The type of juvenile arthritis involving up to four joints is called pauciarticular JA. It usually affects the large joints, such as the knees, ankles, hips, and elbows. It often occurs in just one of a pair of joints; for example, in one knee but not the other.

This form of JA occurs with equal frequency in boys and girls, and it seems to have a peak occurrence when a child is two to three years old. It's less common after age five and rarely occurs after age ten. Inflammation of the eye (covered later in the chapter) is a serious complication of this form of JA.

Juvenile Arthritis (Five or More Joints)

The type of juvenile arthritis involving five or more joints is called polyarticular JA. It usually affects the small joints of the fingers and wrists. It can also affect the weight-bearing joints, including knees, hips, ankles, and feet, along with the neck and jaw. It often affects the same joint on both sides of the body and is accompanied by a low fever. Lumps (rheumatoid nodules) may develop on parts of the body that experience pressure—the elbows, for example.

This form of juvenile arthritis is more common in girls than in boys. It shows up most often between the ages of 2 and 5 and then again between ages 10 and 14. In children under age 10, polyarticular JA often begins with only one or two joints affected; more joints become involved over the next six months.

> **Precautions**
>
> It's always better to be safe than sorry. If a friend or relative says your child's symptoms are just "growing pains," listen to your own instincts and check with your pediatrician.

Systemic Juvenile Arthritis

The type of juvenile arthritis that affects both the joints and the internal organs is called systemic juvenile arthritis. Its symptoms are a fever that comes and goes, a rash, swollen glands, an enlarged liver and spleen, and joint inflammation. It's the least common form of JA. When it occurs after a child turns 16, it's called adult-onset Still's disease.

Systemic JA tends to affect boys and girls in equal numbers, and symptoms usually begin when a child is between three and five years old. Complications, such as inflammation of the heart or of the outer lining of the lungs or heart, are more common with this type of JA. In some cases, systemic JA may progress to polyarticular JA.

What Causes Juvenile Arthritis?

Juvenile arthritis is not contagious. Researchers are working to learn the cause or causes of JA. They know that changes in or abnormalities of the immune system are involved. It's believed that a combination of factors may be responsible.

Genetics

As with many medical conditions, scientists are learning that heredity is an important factor in the development of JA. You may inherit a certain gene that can increase your chances of developing a specific disease, but other factors are probably involved in determining whether the disease actually develops. And though heredity may play a role, it is unusual for more than one child in a family to have juvenile arthritis.

> **Straight Talk**
>
> Find a support group ... the information, education, and support I have gained from my JA buds is priceless. They are there when no one else is!
>
> —Donna, parent, age 40; diagnosed at age 3

The Autoimmune Response

The immune system helps protect the body against disease, fighting off bacterial and viral infections. However, for reasons we do not yet understand, sometimes the system gets confused, breaks down, and begins to fight itself. Then, instead of protecting against disease, it actually creates disease. Certain rheumatic diseases, including certain types of arthritis, are autoimmune diseases.

Bacterial and Viral Infections

A recent bacterial or viral infection may weaken your child's immune system to the point that juvenile arthritis has an opportunity to develop. The infection does not cause JA, but it can contribute to a child developing juvenile arthritis.

Symptoms of Juvenile Arthritis

The most common early symptoms of JA are inflammation of the joints, pain, and fatigue. Joint stiffness, especially after your child has been resting or has been quiet for a while, is also a symptom. A joint may appear swollen, which is often the reason parents make an appointment with the pediatrician. You may notice your child limping, especially in the morning. Your child may or may not complain about pain. These symptoms are fairly typical of early pauciarticular and polyarticular JA.

Systemic JA may cause high spiking fevers that tend to begin in the afternoon or evening. These fevers may continue for weeks or months, but they rarely persist more than six months. A rash that comes and goes, appearing most often on the chest and thighs, accompanies the fever. Chills and shaking may be present, and your child may feel very sick. When you take your child to the pediatrician, blood work will reveal that your child has a very high white blood cell count along with a very low red blood cell count (called anemia).

As juvenile arthritis continues its course, there may be times when the arthritis is particularly active (called flares or flare-ups) and times when symptoms lessen and the joints return to normal. During flares, joints are extremely painful and stiff. Joint damage, *joint contractures*, and changes in growth patterns of the affected joints can occur during these flares.

def•i•ni•tion

A **joint contracture** is a stiff or a bent joint with less than normal range of motion caused by a shortening of the muscle that surrounds the joint. When a child finds it painful to use a joint, the muscle shortens or contracts from lack of use.

Your child may try to relieve the pain of a flare by not using the affected joint; for example, holding her arm in a bent position to avoid using the elbow. Over time, this can cause a contracture. When joint inflammation is severe, the joint surfaces can get worn away. If inflammation damages the growth centers in various bones, a child's growth may slow or stop altogether. Surgery may be needed to correct this.

Diagnosing Juvenile Arthritis

No single test can determine if your child has juvenile arthritis. Arriving at a correct diagnosis can take a little time. At the first office visit, your child's doctor will take your child's health history, conduct a physical exam, perform various lab tests, take some X-rays, and test the fluid in the painful joints. To make a firm diagnosis, the symptoms of JA will usually need to be constantly present for six or more consecutive weeks.

Blood tests are useful in helping make a diagnosis. The nurse or physician assistant will take a small amount of blood. A urinalysis will also be done to see if there are red blood cells, proteins, or other abnormal substances present in the urine. These laboratory tests help your doctor diagnose juvenile arthritis and also help rule out other diseases.

Children may also be affected with arthritis if they have other medical conditions. These include lupus, scleroderma, juvenile dermatomyositis, and certain diseases of the spine.

Your Child's Medical Team

Chapter 8 discusses the roles of the members of an adult's medical support team. Children, however, are not just small adults, and so their care constitutes a special field of medicine, called pediatrics. Some pediatric specialty practices focus on treating children with juvenile arthritis, and if there is one of these practices near where you live, you are fortunate.

As you begin to navigate the health-care system for your child, remember that the most important member of your child's medical team is you, the parent. You may feel unprepared for this task, but be assured—you've got what it takes. In the same way that you learned how to handle all the tasks and responsibilities of parenting, you will learn how to care for your child's arthritis.

First, talk with your child's pediatrician or your family practice physician. Ask questions. Ask for literature so you can read up on JA. The Arthritis Foundation is a wonderful stop in this educational quest. The foundation can provide helpful resources for

Consultation

A spiral notebook with three to five sections is helpful for organizing appointments, medications, questions, concerns, and observations. Choosing one with an attractive cover will make it seem less medical and more user-friendly for both you and your child.

you and may even have a branch office in your area. Check out the foundation's website at www.arthritis.org.

The other essential member of your child's medical team will ideally be a pediatric rheumatologist. Pediatric rheumatologists are pediatricians with additional training in the field of rheumatic diseases, which affect the joints, muscles, bones, skin, and other tissues.

A pediatric rheumatologist has had four years of medical school training, an additional three years of specialization in pediatrics, and an additional two or three years of training in pediatric rheumatology. A pediatric rheumatologist may be board certified by the American Board of Pediatrics.

There is a serious shortage of pediatric rheumatologists, however, and you may have difficulty locating one in your area. The 2007 Pediatric Rheumatology Workforce Report to Congress noted there were fewer than 200 pediatric rheumatologists currently practicing in the United States. Thirteen states have no pediatric rheumatologists at all.

Many major health-care centers have an assortment of specialty practices, including a pediatric rheumatology clinic. Most pediatric rheumatologists, however, practice in academic settings, such as universities, with much of their time spent in research. Finding a pediatric rheumatologist with an active practice who is accepting new patients can be difficult.

Your next best choice is a rheumatologist who treats adult arthritis patients and who may also have experience treating children with juvenile arthritis.

Ask your pediatrician or family practice physician for a referral to a rheumatologist. You can also do some research on your own by checking the American College of Rheumatology's directory at www.rheumatology.org/directory/geo.asp. Another option is your local chapter of the Arthritis Foundation, which can recommend board-certified rheumatologists and pediatric rheumatologists.

Once she has a rheumatologist, your child will be in good hands. If the need for other kinds of doctors or health-care professionals arises, your rheumatologist will refer you, and his office may help you schedule appointments. Who else will be on your child's health-care team?

- **Pediatrician or family practice physician**. Not all of your child's health concerns will be related to juvenile arthritis. You'll still keep in contact with your pediatrician.

- ◆ **Pediatric ophthalmologist.** An ophthalmologist can detect and treat eye inflammation, a complication of one form of JA. (See "Complications" later in this chapter.)

- ◆ **Nurse specialist.** Associated either with the specialty practice or your local hospital, a nurse specialist will explain your child's treatment program in simple language and can answer many of your questions. The specialist is a source for information and resources.

- ◆ **Physical therapist.** A physical therapist will help your child strengthen her muscles and learn how to protect her joints. (See "Physical Therapy" later in this chapter.)

- ◆ **Occupational therapist.** An occupational therapist will help your child learn how to conserve energy while performing daily tasks.

- ◆ **Orthopedist.** Later in the course of JA, your rheumatologist may refer you to an orthopedist, a surgeon specializing in treating bone deformities and performing joint replacements.

- ◆ **Social worker.** A social worker will help your child with strategies for coping with school and with peer relationships.

Medications

Medications are available to treat the symptoms of inflammation and relieve the pain of juvenile arthritis, and research is ongoing to find new and more effective treatments. While there is no cure for JA, early diagnosis and treatment can help provide effective relief for your child's symptoms. Since all drugs have the potential for side effects, periodic urine, blood, and liver function tests will check to be sure everything is normal.

Most of the medications useful for treating arthritis symptoms in adults are also useful for children. Keep in mind that it takes time for many drugs to take effect, sometimes weeks or even months.

Your child's rheumatologist will prescribe the lowest dose that's effective for your child. Even aspirin, a common over-the-counter treatment for JA, may have serious

Precautions

Reye's Syndrome is a rare disease that may occur in children with the flu or chicken pox who are also taking aspirin. If your child contracts the flu or chicken pox, discontinue use of aspirin and contact your pediatrician or rheumatologist.

side effects in children. Remember also that all drugs should be kept out of the reach of children. An overdose can be fatal.

See Chapter 9 for an in-depth discussion of both over-the-counter and prescription drugs used for treating the symptoms of arthritis.

Nonsurgical Treatments

If medication and other nonsurgical approaches are helpful in treating your child's symptoms, surgery may be postponed or avoided altogether.

Physical Therapy

Physical therapy (PT) is one of these very important nonsurgical approaches. Many physical therapists work with children and understand their special needs and concerns. Physical therapy can teach your child how to protect her joints and also how to conserve her energy both at school and at home.

The physical therapist will work with your child to strengthen the muscles that surround the joints affected with JA. This strengthening will encourage your child to use those joints and help avoid contractures. (See Chapter 17 for more information on specific exercises used in physical therapy.)

One complication of juvenile arthritis is uneven leg length, which we'll discuss later in this chapter. This can throw off your child's gait. Your child's physical therapist can prescribe inserts for your child's shoes that will help correct this problem.

Assistive Devices

The physical therapist can fit your child with assistive devices to hold the joints in the proper position and provide additional support. These assistive devices include knee extension splints, wrist extension splints, and ring splints for the fingers, all in sizes made for children's smaller joints.

A splint is used when a child's joint is in danger of becoming deformed or is already showing signs of deformity. The splint may be used to gradually stretch and return the joint to its normal position. These splints are constructed and fitted by an occupational or physical therapist and are usually only worn at night, while your child is sleeping. During the day, your child may wear a functional splint, called an orthosis or brace, which allows some joint movement but still offers support.

Surgical Treatments

Surgery is not usually necessary during the earlier stages of JA. If your rheumatologist agrees that surgery is indicated, however, there are three procedures that are commonly performed.

Removing the Inflamed Joint Lining

This procedure is called synovectomy. It removes the inflamed joint lining tissue, called the synovium. Removing the diseased tissue can relieve the pain of juvenile arthritis. It's done on the knees most frequently, but elbows, wrists, and shoulders can also be candidates for this procedure.

Joint Replacement

Older, physically mature children who have severe joint damage are the best candidates to have a joint replaced with an artificial joint. In children who are still growing, joint size is changing, as well. Hip, knee, and jaw joints are most frequently replaced. The surgery can relieve your child's pain and also increase the affected joint's range of motion and functionality.

The main reason joint replacement surgery isn't done on younger children is that these artificial joints eventually wear out and require replacement. A second replacement surgery is more involved and may have more potential for complications. Since the life span for an artificial hip or knee joint is 10 to 20 years with current technology, it's possible your child will need several of these joint replacements over her lifetime. Researchers are working on new joint replacement materials that have longer life spans and will reduce the number of additional surgeries needed.

Soft Tissue Release

Soft tissue release improves a joint contracture by lengthening the tendons. The surgeon cuts the tissues that caused the contracture and then repairs them. This allows the joint to return to its normal position.

Complications

The more serious complications of JA include chronic eye inflammation and vision problems for children with pauciarticular JA and specific joint problems or decreased growth for children with polyarticular or systemic JA.

Eye Inflammation

Two kinds of eye inflammation can occur as complications of pauciarticular JA. The first is iridocyclitis, an inflammation of the iris and the ciliary body—two structures within the eye. The second is anterior uveitis (iritis), inflammation of the front part of the uveal tract, which lines the inside of the eye behind the cornea. Anterior uveitis affects approximately 20 to 25 percent of children with pauciarticular JA.

Young girls with pauciarticular JA are most likely to develop iridocyclitis if their blood contains a kind of protein known as an antinuclear antibody (ANA). A child below the age of 6 with this marker has an increased risk of developing uveitis.

There are frequently no early symptoms for these very serious complications, and even with therapy, more than 15 percent of children with chronic uveitis suffer permanent damage to their vision.

Regular screenings by an ophthalmologist are important to detect and treat these conditions and help prevent permanent damage to your child's vision. Keeping track of changes in your child's eyes will help your ophthalmologist deal with these potential complications. A procedure called a slit-lamp eye examination uses magnified 3-D imagery to view the different parts of the eye. Special lenses can be placed between the lamp and the cornea or even directly on the cornea to look at structures deep in the eye. A camera attached to the lamp takes pictures of the entire procedure.

Eyedrops are most often used to treat these conditions, but if they aren't effective, your ophthalmologist may prescribe medication in pill form.

Uneven Leg Length

When the knee joint becomes inflamed, blood flow to that joint increases. The blood carries nutrients with it and those nutrients cause the joint to overgrow—often in length as well as in width. Over time, this overgrowth can become noticeable. Injection of a steroid, such as cortisone, into the joint early in the course of JA may prevent this from occurring.

If the difference in length between the affected leg and the healthy leg is less than one centimeter, surgery is usually not indicated. In these cases, placing a lift inside one shoe evens things out. However, if the difference is greater than one centimeter, the child's gait is affected, and eventually hip problems can occur.

In cases where the discrepancy in leg length is enough to point toward surgery, you'll schedule a consultation with an orthopedic surgeon before your child reaches *skeletal maturity*. If he advises surgery, he'll staple the growth plate of the tibia in the longer leg to allow the opposite leg to catch up. This is considered minor surgery and generally produces good results.

def•i•ni•tion

When the bones reach **skeletal maturity,** they have achieved maximum growth. A doctor uses X-ray imagery of the bones to discover their developmental stage and determine whether skeletal maturity has been reached.

Jaw Malformation

The joint just in front of the ears, where the lower jaw connects to the skull, is called the temporomandibular joint. This joint can be affected by arthritis, which causes pain, stiffness, and changes in normal growth patterns.

Your dentist needs to be aware of your child's diagnosis of juvenile arthritis. This will help her provide the best care possible and be alert for any significant changes that develop in your child's jaw. She may prescribe jaw exercises, along with heat and cold therapy, to relieve pain and discomfort.

If the lower jaw is not developing properly, your child may develop a severe overbite. If this happens, your dentist will refer you to an orthodontist for consultation and treatment. Surgery may be necessary to correct this condition. Your dentist may also prescribe an antibiotic for your child to take before any dental work is performed to decrease chances of infection. Always inform your dentist of all medications your child is taking.

Precautions

Keep a list handy of all medications your child is taking. Your spiral notebook is the best place to keep track. If any new medication is prescribed, be sure to ask the pharmacist about any possible drug interactions.

Prognosis Concerns

When your child is first diagnosed with juvenile arthritis, all kinds of questions and concerns arise. You want to know what this will mean for your child and for your family. You want to know if there's a cure. Unfortunately, right now, there isn't, though many of the symptoms of JA can be effectively treated. Researchers continue to seek both the cause and the cure and hopefully, before too much longer, we'll know both.

Consultation _____

Up to 80 percent of children affected by JA regain normal joint function by age 16. At least half the children with pauciarticular JA and slightly less than half the children with polyarticular JA experience a complete remission of their symptoms.

Your child's prognosis depends to a great extent upon the type of JA she has, the quality of care she receives, whether or not she develops complications, and the age at which her symptoms began. Children who show symptoms before they are five years old have the most serious prognosis, but the course of JA is different in each child, which makes generalizations very difficult. Overall, though, the prognosis is good.

Of the three types of juvenile arthritis, pauciarticular JA has the best prognosis, although one fourth of these children experience long-term complications related to their eyes. These complications can include reduced vision, cataracts, glaucoma, or blindness.

The prognosis for systemic JA depends a great deal on the organs involved and whether or not the disease progresses to polyarticular JA. More than half of these children go into remission and never have another recurrence of their symptoms.

Polyarticular JA has a difficult prognosis, with the possibility of serious joint deformity and the eventual need for total joint replacement surgeries.

Juvenile arthritis is a chronic disease, but chronic doesn't necessarily mean permanent, and it's important to remember that JA can go into remission—meaning that the symptoms all go away—at any time. Doctors do not know yet how this happens. Remission can last for several months or years or forever. With proper therapy, a nutritious diet, exercise, and the right medications, your child has a good chance of getting well with no serious, permanent disabilities.

The Least You Need to Know

◆ Juvenile arthritis is the most common type of arthritis affecting children under age 16.

◆ The main types of juvenile arthritis are pauciarticular, polyarticular, and systemic.

◆ The types of juvenile arthritis are defined by the number of joints involved and whether or not certain organs of the body are affected.

- Pediatric rheumatologists are uniquely trained to help children with JA, but there is a serious shortage of these physicians. Many adult rheumatologists also treat children, particularly in areas without a pediatric rheumatologist.

- Medication, physical therapy, and surgery are treatment options for JA. The primary focus of treatment is on relieving pain and preventing joint damage and complications.

- The prognosis for JA is largely a factor of which subtype your child has. Remission is possible at any time.

Chapter 6

Arthritis of the Spine, Joints, Ligaments, and Tendons

In This Chapter

- Beyond simple joint pain
- Understanding ankylosing spondylitis
- What is psoriatic arthritis?
- How reactive arthritis develops
- About enteropathic arthritis

The inflammatory arthritic conditions affecting the spine, joints, ligaments, and tendons are known as the spondyloarthropies. These forms of arthritis can lead to serious complications, including spinal deformity and damage to the heart valves. As with other types of arthritis, there is no cure for the spondyloarthropies, and treatment centers around slowing the progress of the disease and relieving pain.

Ankylosing Spondylitis

Ankylosing spondylitis (AS) affects the joints and the ligaments of the spine. It also impacts your sacroiliac joints, which are located where the bone directly above your tailbone (sacrum) meets the bones on either side of your upper buttocks (iliac bones). AS is a systemic disease, which means it can affect other tissues throughout your body, causing inflammation in the eyes, heart, lungs, and kidneys.

Symptoms of AS can range from mild to severe. Your spine may be painful and stiff. Over time, chronic inflammation of the spine can result in the spine fusing together, making it rigid. This fusing is called *ankylosis* and gives AS its name.

The pain goes away once the spine has fused—that's the good part. The bad part is that the spine then can't move. It becomes brittle and prone to fractures in the event of a fall or an accident. This fusing process may progress more slowly in women than in men, meaning that women may experience pain for a longer period of time.

Precautions

If you have advanced ankylosing spondylitis and experience a sudden onset of pain along with increased mobility in the spine, you may have sustained a fracture. This is usually associated with a fall or auto accident. The lower neck, called the cervical spine, is the most common site for these fractures. Go to an emergency room or check with your rheumatologist to rule out this possibility.

AS generally progresses slowly, and early diagnosis and treatment are essential to help control symptoms and reduce spinal deformity. With proper care, most people with AS can continue to live and work normally.

Symptoms

Symptoms of ankylosing spondylitis often begin in late adolescence or early adulthood. Each person tends to have a unique pattern of symptoms and disease activity. Early symptoms are pain and stiffness in the buttocks and lower back, moving up the spine to involve the chest and neck.

Generally, symptoms progress gradually, but they can occasionally be acute and intense. Shoulders and hips can also be involved, as can tendons and ligaments. You can develop Achilles tendonitis or pain in your heel (plantar fasciitis). Fatigue and fever can also be symptoms.

Pain and stiffness are usually worse in the morning or after periods of prolonged inactivity. Motion, heat, and a warm shower can ease these symptoms.

Breathing difficulties are also symptoms of AS. If AS involves areas where your ribs attach to your upper spine, it can affect your lung capacity. Also, as AS progresses, the upper body may curve forward, making breathing difficult. Since AS may cause inflammation and scarring of the lungs, coughing and shortness of breath may become a problem, especially while exercising. Fortunately, this is a rare complication of AS.

If your eyes become inflamed, you may have pain in your eyes, especially when looking at bright light. These attacks of inflammation may come and go and may affect either eye. This inflammation should be promptly evaluated and treated by an ophthalmologist to prevent vision loss.

In very rare cases, the heart's electrical system can become scarred, resulting in an abnormally slow heart rate. A pacemaker may be necessary to correct this problem. If the part of the aorta closest to the heart becomes inflamed, the aortic valve may leak. Shortness of breath, dizziness, and heart failure can result.

In rare advanced cases of AS, deposits of protein material, called amyloid, may occur in the kidneys, resulting in kidney failure. If the kidney disease progresses, dialysis or transplantation may be necessary.

> **Precautions**
>
> Cigarette smoking can increase lung scarring and breathing difficulties in people with AS. If you smoke, quitting is one of the best things you can do.

Who Gets Ankylosing Spondylitis?

Ankylosing spondylitis affects 1 in 1,000 people. It's more common in Caucasians than in other racial groups and usually more severe in males than in females. AS can affect all age groups although it is rare for AS to begin after age 45. It usually affects people in their teens, 20s, and 30s.

Causes

The specific cause or causes of AS aren't yet known, but genetics may be involved. Nearly 90 percent of people with AS have a specific gene, known as HLA-B27. About 7 percent of the population of the United States has this gene, but only 1 percent

Consultation

HLA-B27-positive individuals with relatives who have AS are six times more likely to develop this disease than those whose relatives do not have AS.

actually develops ankylosing spondylitis. Recent research has identified two additional genes associated with AS. These genes seem to play a role in influencing immune function.

Other factors in addition to these genes, such as bacterial infections, may be involved in determining whether the disease develops. An infection activates the body's immune system, but after the infection has cleared up, the immune system may not turn off. Instead, it may turn on the body itself, mistaking it for a foreign invader.

Diagnosis

Stiffness and lower back pain are symptoms associated with many medical conditions, and it may take some time to arrive at a diagnosis of ankylosing spondylitis. In adolescents, lower back pain may be thought to be a result of sports-related injuries.

As with other types of arthritic conditions, a diagnosis begins with a careful history, physical examination, X-rays, and blood tests. X-rays or even MRI of the sacroiliac joints may be helpful. There is no blood test to detect AS, and the presence of the HLA-B27 gene by itself can't confirm or rule out AS. Urinalysis can look for kidney abnormalities and may be used to exclude kidney conditions that cause lower back pain.

Treatment

It's important to seek treatment early for the best prognosis. Because AS is an inflammatory disease, treatment focuses on reducing inflammation and suppressing the overactive immune system. Physical therapy and exercise are also important to help prevent spinal deformity and increase spinal mobility and lung capacity.

Precautions

Taking these medications with food can help minimize side effects, which can include stomach upset, nausea, abdominal pain, and diarrhea.

Medications used to treat AS include aspirin and other nonsteroidal anti-inflammatory drugs (NSAIDs). Commonly used NSAIDs include indomethacin (Indocin), tolmetin (Tolectin), sulindac (Clinoril), naproxen (Naprosyn), and diclofenac (Voltaren).

NSAIDs are effective in reducing inflammation but don't change the natural history of the disease.

When symptoms extend beyond the spine and inflammation occurs in the hips, knees, or ankles, medications that suppress the immune system may then be added. These medications may include sulfasalazine (Azulfidine), leflunomide (Arava), and most frequently methotrexate (Rheumatrex, Trexall), which can be administered orally or by injection. If your rheumatologist prescribes methotrexate or other DMARDs for you, you will have periodic blood tests to keep tabs on your liver and bone marrow functions, to safeguard against cirrhosis and anemia.

Importantly, while traditional DMARDs may control joint symptoms in the extremities, they are not effective for the spinal arthritis. Fortunately, newer medications, referred to as biologics, have been quite effective in treating both peripheral joint and spinal arthritis of ankylosing spondylitis. Called TNF (tumor necrosis factor) blockers, they stop disease activity, decrease inflammation, and improve spinal mobility. Examples of these TNF blockers include etanercept (Enbrel), infliximab (Remicade), and adalimumab (Humira). Improvement can be sustained over a period of years with continued use of these biologics. The biologics are given as IVs in the doctor's office or by self-administered shots at home.

Cortisone eyedrops may be necessary to treat inflammation of the iris of the eyes. Rarely, high doses of cortisone administered orally may be necessary. Atropine eyedrops can be useful to relax the muscles of the iris. If inflammation is severe, cortisone injections into the eye may be required.

Surgical options to treat AS are limited. When AS is severe, shoulder or hip replacement may help. In rare instances, spinal osteotomy can be performed to reduce the forward curvature of the spine.

Physical therapy (PT) is an essential component of a treatment program for ankylosing spondylitis. Maintaining an erect posture is important, and PT can give you stretching exercises and back extension exercises to improve the mobility of your spine and joints. If you have AS, you should sleep on a firm mattress and avoid the use of a pillow in order to prevent spine curvature. PT can also teach you deep breathing exercises to expand your lungs.

Aerobic exercise promotes full expansion of the breathing muscles and opens the airways of the lungs. You should avoid jarring your spine, so swimming is an excellent choice for exercise. Try to stand, walk, and sit tall at all times.

Consultation

If you are pregnant or considering becoming pregnant, you should know that AS has no harmful effect on the course of pregnancy or on fetal well-being. Compared to healthy women, however, women with AS are more likely to undergo a cesarean section.

Prognosis

Ankylosing spondylitis is a chronic disease, but rarely a fatal one. Most people with AS lead normal lives. Medication combined with physical exercise can help keep your symptoms under control.

Psoriatic Arthritis

When inflammatory arthritis exists along with psoriasis, the condition is known as psoriatic arthritis. There are several types of psoriatic arthritis, with symptoms that range from mild to severe.

Psoriasis is a familiar skin condition that affects about 2 percent of the Caucasian population of the United States. Patchy, raised, red, and scaly skin are characteristics of psoriasis, which often affects the tips of the elbows and knees, the scalp, the navel, and the area around the genitals or anus. Approximately 10 percent of people with psoriasis also develop inflammation of their joints. Fingernails and toenails can become pitted and discolored.

Psoriatic arthritis.

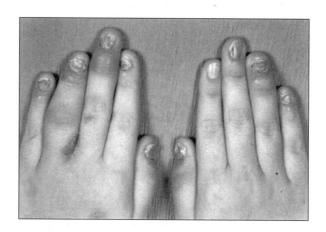

Psoriatic arthritis isn't generally as crippling as rheumatoid arthritis, but without treatment it can cause discomfort, disability, and deformity. Medication, physical therapy, and lifestyle changes can often relieve pain and slow joint damage. There are several different types of psoriatic arthritis.

Asymmetric Arthritis

This is the mildest type of psoriatic arthritis. Because it's asymmetrical, it affects certain joints on one side of your body or different joints on both sides of your body. There's no specific pattern to which joints are involved. Usually one to three joints are affected; these tend to be the wrist, hip, knee, or ankle. If you have asymmetric arthritis in your hands or feet, you may notice that your fingers or toes take on the appearance of little sausages. This is because of swelling and inflammation in the tendons.

Symmetric Arthritis

This type of psoriatic arthritis is similar to rheumatoid arthritis. Because it's symmetrical, it tends to affect the same joints on both sides of the body. It can involve four or more joints. Women tend to have this type of psoriatic arthritis more than men, and the psoriasis can be severe.

Distal Interphalangeal Joint Predominant (DIP)

This type of psoriatic arthritis tends to affect the small joints nearest the fingernails and toenails, causing problems with these nails. DIP affects more men than women and sometimes is mistaken for osteoarthritis.

Arthritis Mutilans

This is a very painful and crippling type of psoriatic arthritis. Over time, it can actually destroy the small bones of the hand, especially in the fingers.

Psoriatic Spondylitis

This type of psoriatic arthritis causes spinal inflammation and stiffness and inflammation from the neck to the lower back's sacroiliac joints. It's not quite the same condition as ankylosing spondylitis.

Symptoms

Symptoms of psoriatic arthritis can come and go and the symptoms of psoriasis may not occur at the same time as the symptoms of arthritis. Joint stiffness is common and is typically worse early in the morning. Knees, ankles, and joints in the feet are often affected, although usually only a few joints are inflamed at one time. Sometimes joint inflammation in the fingers or toes can cause swelling of the entire digit, giving it a sausage-like appearance.

In many people, the symptoms of psoriasis occur long before the symptoms of arthritis, although some people experience joint pain before they develop psoriasis. To be diagnosed with psoriatic arthritis, you must show symptoms of both psoriasis and arthritis.

Psoriatic arthritis can develop slowly and have mild symptoms, or it can develop quickly and be severe. The National Psoriasis Foundation advises that early recognition, diagnosis, and treatment can help prevent or limit the extensive joint damage that occurs in later stages of the disease.

Who Gets Psoriatic Arthritis?

Psoriatic arthritis may affect as many as one million of the approximately six million Americans who have psoriasis. Most are adults in their 30s, 40s, and 50s; however, children can also develop a form of the disease. The National Psoriasis Foundation Benchmark Survey found that Caucasians were more likely to develop psoriatic arthritis than African Americans. For more information, check out the foundation's website at www.psoriasis.org.

Causes

According to the Mayo Clinic (www.mayoclinic.com), having psoriasis is the single greatest risk factor for psoriatic arthritis. Your chances also increase if you have a family member with psoriatic arthritis. As with other types of arthritis, a combination of genetic and environmental factors determine whether or not you develop psoriatic arthritis.

Other risk factors for psoriatic arthritis include skin injuries, strep infections, stress, alcohol abuse, poor nutrition, or a reaction to medications or vaccinations.

Diagnosis

Diagnosis of psoriatic arthritis can be time-consuming and difficult. You're considered to have psoriatic arthritis only when you have symptoms of both psoriasis and arthritis. You may develop arthritis before you develop psoriasis and vice versa. It's even possible to have joint pain—from osteoarthritis, for example—with psoriasis and not have psoriatic arthritis.

No single test can confirm a diagnosis of psoriatic arthritis, although certain tests can help distinguish psoriatic arthritis from other conditions. X-rays, for example, can reveal changes in the joints that occur in psoriatic arthritis but not in other arthritic conditions; joint fluid analysis can be used to rule out gout; and blood tests can determine if you have rheumatoid factor or anti-CCP antibody (often present with rheumatoid arthritis) or anemia (a common condition in people with psoriatic arthritis).

Treatment

The goals of treatment are to reduce joint pain and swelling, slow or prevent joint damage, and relieve dry, scaling skin. Your doctor is likely to prescribe a combination of medication, exercise, and physical therapy.

For mild psoriatic arthritis, your doctor may recommend nonsteroidal anti-inflammatory drugs (NSAIDs), such as aspirin and ibuprofen (Advil, Motrin), or a COX-2 inhibitor, such as celecoxib (Celebrex), to help control pain, swelling, and morning stiffness. NSAIDs generally don't help psoriasis, and some may even make skin problems worse. Still, these medications may be a good option for people with minor joint pain and stiffness.

Other prescription options include one of the disease-modifying antirheumatic drugs (DMARDs). Examples of DMARDs include sulfasalazine (Azulfidine), the antimalarial drug hydroxychloroquine (Plaquenil), and methotrexate (Rheumatrex). Of these agents, methotrexate is by far the most commonly used, as it improves the symptoms of both psoriasis and psoriatic arthritis.

Tumor necrosis factor (TNF) blockers are used to slow or prevent permanent joint damage. These blockers are biologics that block an immune system protein called tumor necrosis factor, which causes inflammation in some types of arthritis. TNF blockers provide pain relief, reduce joint swelling, and ease stiffness. Three TNF blockers approved for treating psoriatic arthritis are etanercept (Enbrel), adalimumab (Humira), and infliximab (Remicade).

Because of their side effects, corticosteroids are generally prescribed for the shortest amount of time necessary and in the smallest doses effective.

Your dermatologist will treat the symptoms of psoriasis with oral medications, topical creams and ointments, or ultraviolet light or sunlight therapy (phototherapy). Because

Consultation

It can take some time for DMARDs to take effect. In the meantime, your rheumatologist may prescribe a pain reliever (such as aspirin) in addition to a DMARD.

no two people have the exact same symptoms, your treatment plan will be tailored to your specific needs.

Prognosis

Until recently, psoriatic arthritis had been considered a milder disease than rheumatoid arthritis, but new evidence is showing that this may not be true. To decrease the chance of disability and physical deformity, early diagnosis and treatment of psoriatic arthritis is essential.

Reactive Arthritis (Reiter's Syndrome)

Reactive arthritis develops as the result of an infection. It affects the joints of the spine and the sacroiliac (the area where the spine attaches to the pelvis). It can also affect other parts of the body, including the arms and legs. Reactive arthritis was once called Reiter's Syndrome.

Consultation _____

Reiter's Syndrome was named for Dr. Hans Reiter. He was a German military physician who, during World War I, treated a lieutenant with bloody diarrhea and a high fever who went on to develop arthritis, conjunctivitis, and urethritis. Reiter's authorization of medical experiments in Nazi concentration camps during World War II has caused his name to fall out of favor, and the disease is now called _reactive arthritis,_ a term first used in 1967.

Symptoms

Reactive arthritis usually begins with an intestinal or urinary tract infection. It's characterized by inflammation of the joints, urinary tract, and eyes, in addition to mouth and skin ulcers. The symptoms usually begin one to four weeks after the initial infection and they may appear gradually or develop quickly. The symptoms include fever, weight loss, skin rash, sores, and pain, though the symptoms tend to come and go and to not occur at the same time. Not everyone with reactive arthritis experiences all of these symptoms.

Reactive arthritis is often asymmetric, which means it affects different joints on opposite sides of the body and usually affects a small number of joints. Each episode may involve different joints. There may be inflammation in the areas where tendons connect to the bones, such as in the ankles and heels.

A small percentage of people have constant and continuing joint involvement. In most cases, however, symptoms stop after three to six months. For about half the people who have an attack of reactive arthritis, the first attack is the only one. If you do have a second bout, your odds of not having a third attack are again 50 percent. However, if the attacks continue, it becomes more likely that the disease will become chronic. In most cases, reactive arthritis does not lead to permanent joint damage or disability.

Who Gets Reactive Arthritis?

Reactive arthritis is most common in Caucasian men between the ages of 20 and 40. About 4,500 cases are identified each year in the United States. African American males rarely get reactive arthritis, and women get it one fifth as frequently as men.

Causes

Although the exact cause is unknown, reactive arthritis tends to run in some families, which may indicate a genetic link. A gene marker called HLA-B27 is present in about 75 percent of people who develop reactive arthritis.

Reactive arthritis may develop following an intestinal, genital, or urinary tract infection. It usually occurs through inflammation of the intestinal tract followed by a bout of diarrhea caused by eating foods contaminated with bacteria, such as salmonella. Exactly how joints and other organs become involved after the initial infection is not known.

Studies show that some people develop reactive arthritis or have a relapse after having sexual intercourse with a new partner, probably due to reaction to infection with chlamydia.

Diagnosis

Reactive arthritis is diagnosed with detailed history, particularly of a preceding gastrointestinal or genitourinary infection, a physical exam, and a test for the presence of the HLA-B27 gene. This diagnostic period can take some time, especially if you do not show all the symptoms at once. Generally, the more symptoms present, the quicker the diagnosis. Your doctor will expect to see arthritis that predominantly involves the lower limbs, involves few joints, and involves one side of the body more than the other.

Treatment

The goal of treatment is to reduce inflammation and treat any existing infection. Medications such as nonsteroidal anti-inflammatory drugs (NSAIDs), antibiotics, and topical skin preparations are used, along with eyedrops. For individuals with severe or persistent symptoms, DMARDs and even biologic agents may be necessary to control the disease. Joint protection may also be necessary.

Because of the differing nature of the symptoms, a variety of health-care professionals may be involved in your treatment. Your rheumatologist will refer you to the necessary specialists and coordinate your treatment plan. A dermatologist will treat skin lesions, an ophthalmologist will treat eye problems, and a urologist will treat problems with your urinary tract.

Prognosis

Within two to six months, most people with reactive arthritis experience a full recovery. In some cases, arthritis symptoms may persist for up to a year, although they tend to be mild. In about 20 percent of cases, the arthritis becomes chronic, although it usually is not disabling.

Enteropathic Arthritis

The Spondylitis Organization of America describes enteropathic arthritis as a form of chronic, inflammatory arthritis associated with inflammatory bowel disease (IBD). About one in five people with IBD will develop enteropathic arthritis.

The arm and leg joints are most commonly affected by enteropathic arthritis. In some cases, the entire spine can become inflamed as well. Up to 50 percent of people with enteropathic arthritis with spine involvement have the HLA-B27 gene.

Symptoms

The symptoms of enteropathic arthritis can be divided into symptoms of IBD and arthritic symptoms in the joints and possibly elsewhere. Symptoms of arthritis and IBD generally occur at the same time. Controlling the IBD usually leads to improvement of the peripheral joint symptoms.

Arthritis symptoms usually begin after IBD has become chronic. Enteropathic arthritis is not usually disabling.

Who Gets Enteropathic Arthritis?

Enteropathic arthritis is most common in young adults and adolescents. It affects males and females equally, and it is seen in 10 to 20 percent of people with IBD.

Causes

The exact cause of enteropathic arthritis is unknown. In people with IBD, the intestine is constantly inflamed. This inflammation may permit bacteria to gain entrance through the bowel wall and enter the bloodstream. Sores on the skin, and joint, spinal, and eye inflammation can result.

Diagnosis

A diagnosis is made through a complete medical examination, including a history of symptoms and a family history. A stool sample may be taken if a diagnosis of an IBD, such as ulcerative colitis or Crohn's disease, has not yet been established. A colonoscopy with or without bowel biopsies may also be done.

Blood tests may be done to detect inflammation or the presence of the HLA-B27 genetic marker. Joint fluid may be taken for analysis, along with X-rays of the affected joints.

Treatment

A number of different types of medication are effective in managing the symptoms of inflammatory bowel disease and enteropathic arthritis. Your rheumatologist may work with a gastroenterologist to help treat the IBD. A gastroenterologist is a physician who specializes in diseases of the gastrointestinal tract.

Nonsteroidal anti-inflammatory drugs (NSAIDs) are commonly used to treat arthritis symptoms but can irritate the intestinal lining and actually intensify the inflammation.

Injection of steroids into the affected joints can be very helpful. Oral steroids can be used in more severe cases. In resistant cases, medications normally used to treat rheumatoid arthritis, such as methotrexate (Rheumatrex, Trexall), azathioprine (Imuran), or sulfasalazine (Azulfidine), can be tried. Adalimumab (Humira) and infliximab (Remicade) may also be prescribed, as they provide very effective relief of both the inflammatory bowel disease and the associated arthritis.

Prognosis

The symptoms of enteropathic arthritis vary from person to person and so does the course of the disease itself. Recurrences are common. While there is no cure at the present time, medications and other therapies can provide relief of both arthritis and IBD.

The Least You Need to Know

◆ Maintaining good posture can help prevent spinal deformity with ankylosing spondylitis.

◆ Some types of arthritis can develop in the aftermath of a bacterial infection.

◆ When tissues and organs are involved, arthritis is considered to be systemic.

◆ Early diagnosis and treatment of arthritis is essential for a good prognosis.

Chapter 7

Gout and Pseudogout

In This Chapter

- The "rich man's arthritis"?
- Who is affected?
- Causes and risk factors
- The signs and symptoms of gout
- Diagnosis and treatment options
- Pseudogout: "false gout"

Gout and pseudogout are types of crystalline arthritis, the form of arthritis that conjures up pictures of an elderly rich man, sitting in an easy chair with an elevated, bandaged foot. It's a classic case of blaming the patient for overindulgence in rich food and strong drink. While the picture may be humorous, gout and pseudogout are forms of chronic arthritis that are not humorous at all.

What Is Gout?

Gout has the rather dubious distinction of being one of history's most frequently recorded and discussed ailments. Although traditionally it's been associated with consumption of too much rich food and alcohol—the wealthy man's arthritis—the reality is that anyone can develop gout, although certain foods may indeed trigger an outbreak.

Gout usually affects only one or two joints at a time and the feet and ankles are prime targets. Gout comes on quickly, often overnight, and the sudden onset of pain can be excruciating. The classic area affected is the first tarsometatarsal joint where the big toe attaches to the foot, and the swelling that results can cause the skin over the affected joint to become red and shiny.

This first attack subsides in a week or so. Early on in the course of gout, there can be an interval of months or even years between attacks. Eventually, attacks tend to become more frequent and more severe, and many joints may be involved with each attack. At this point, the gout is considered to have become chronic, and progressive joint damage can result.

Straight Talk

Persons affected with the gout who are aged, have tophi (crystals) in their joints, who have led a hard life, and whose bowels are constipated are beyond the power of medicine to cure.

—Hippocratic writings (about 400 B.C.E.)

Who Gets Gout?

It's estimated that 1 to 3 million people in the United States suffer from attacks of gout. This condition and its complications occur most often in men, women who have gone through menopause particularly if taking diuretics, and people with kidney disease. The American College of Rheumatology notes that the prevalence of gout has risen substantially over the last two decades in the United States, rising particularly rapidly among the elderly and in postmenopausal women.

If you suffer from gout, and *suffer* is definitely the right word, you're in good historical company. Both Henry VIII and Benjamin Franklin had terrible gout. Franklin even wrote a comic dialogue with "Madam Gout" which he dated "midnight, 22 October, 1780." The gout was keeping him awake. He is quoted as saying "Be temperate in wine, in eating, girls, and cloth, or the Gout will seize you and plague you both."

There is a tendency for gout to run in families, and this may indicate a genetic factor at work. Your body's inability to process uric acid properly may be an inherited trait.

What Causes Gout?

Gout develops when uric acid, which is a normal waste product, isn't excreted efficiently. When everything is functioning normally, uric acid dissolves in your bloodstream and passes through your kidneys into your urine.

When there's a problem—your body creating too much uric acid or your kidneys failing to excrete all the uric acid that passes into them, for example—uric acid levels in your body rise and sharp, needle-like crystals are deposited in and around your joints. These crystals may attract white blood cells, which can lead to severe inflammation. When these crystals are deposited in the urinary tract, they can cause kidney stones to develop.

When gout becomes chronic, nodules (tophi) of uric acid crystals can deposit in soft tissues in different parts of your body. Mostly these nodules appear around your fingers, the tips of your elbows, and around your big toe, although they can appear anywhere. In some cases nodules have been found in the ears, on the vocal cords, and—rarely—around the spinal column.

In addition to genetics, other risk factors for gout include obesity, moderate to heavy alcohol use, diuretics prescribed for heart failure or high blood pressure, and abnormal kidney function. Dehydration, injury to a joint, fever, excessive eating, and recent surgery can also put you at risk for developing gout.

> **Consultation**
>
> To decrease your risk of gout attacks, keep hydrated by drinking plenty of water, especially when the heat and humidity rise.

It's believed that gout attacks triggered by recent surgery may be related to changes in your body's fluid balance. This balance can be upset when you follow the pre-surgery requirement of not taking in fluids a certain number of hours before surgery.

Medications, particularly thiazide and other diuretics, as well as high doses of aspirin, niacin, cyclosporine, and medications for treating tuberculosis (pyrazinamide and ethambutol), may lead to gout by raising blood uric acid levels.

Certain medical conditions, such as leukemia, lymphoma, and hemoglobin disorders, can also cause your body to produce excess uric acid. Having diabetes or high blood pressure can also put you at increased risk for gout.

A complicated chain of medical events can increase your risk of developing gout. For example, having metabolic syndrome puts you at risk for developing diabetes.

Also known as syndrome X, metabolic syndrome is a cluster of factors that increase risk of disease. These factors include high blood pressure, cholesterol abnormalities, increased risk of clotting, insulin resistance, and abdominal obesity. Insulin resistance means that your body's cells have a diminished ability to respond to the action of insulin in promoting the transport of glucose from blood into muscles and other tissues. Insulin resistance also promotes excessive uric acid, a condition known as hyperuricemia. Excessive uric acid can lead to gout.

The Weather Connection

Can you blame gout on the weather? Surprisingly, that's a possibility! According to research presented at the American College of Rheumatology Annual Scientific Meeting, heat and humidity can lead to dehydration, and dehydration can bring on an attack of gout.

For this study, researchers recruited 197 people who had had an attack of gout within the past year. Using an online questionnaire, participants logged on when they experienced an attack and were asked to report on the risk factors they had experienced over a two-day period before the attack began—a time the researchers dubbed "the hazard period." They also completed the same questionnaire over a two-day period when they did not subsequently have a gout attack. Information on alcohol intake, use of diuretics, and *purine* intake were factored in.

def•i•ni•tion

A **purine** is a white crystalline substance that's one of the building blocks of DNA. When purine is broken down in the body as part of the metabolic process, it creates uric acid.

Using National Oceanic and Atmospheric Administration data on temperature, barometric pressure, humidity, and precipitation for both the hazard period and the control period, researchers determined that high temperatures and high humidity were strongly associated with increased risk for recurrences of gout.

In fact, the risk increased almost twofold when the maximum daily temperature increased from 0–53°F to 87–105°F. Risk also increased when the humidity increased from the dew point of 4–32°F to 64–77°F.

Alcohol, Meat, Seafood, and Gout

What you eat can have an impact on whether or not you develop gout. Increased meat and seafood consumption, along with decreased consumption of dairy foods, has been linked to higher levels of uric acid, which can lead to gout. The Health Professionals Study was a 12-year study conducted at Harvard Medical School that involved more than 47,000 male medical professionals aged 40 and older who did not have gout at the beginning of the study. At the follow-up to the study, 730 cases of gout had developed, and these developed among those who had the highest consumption of meat and seafood. Those who regularly consumed low-fat dairy products, such as yogurt and skim milk, lowered their risk of gout.

The Health Professionals Study also found that even moderate regular consumption of beer was associated with a high risk of developing gout, while moderate consumption of wine (1–2 glasses per day) was not.

Is it the alcohol, or is it just beer that can lead to attacks of gout? Part of it is the diuretic, dehydrating effects of alcohol. Alcohol also can increase uric acid production. This twofold effect of slowing down the excretion of uric acid from the kidneys, along with dehydration, can cause uric acid crystals to form in the joints.

It's important to understand that not everyone with elevated levels of uric acid develops gout, and likewise, not everyone with gout has elevated levels of uric acid. It is possible to have gout with normal or even low uric acid levels. In the United States, about 10 percent of men have elevated uric acid levels. Only a small number of these men will ever develop gout.

While overall alcohol consumption per capita in the United States has declined over the past 20 years, consumption of beer, and particularly "light beers," has grown. Light or not, beer is still beer. So what's in beer that increases your chances of developing gout? Purines. Beer has a high purine content.

Precautions

A combination of factors most likely determines if you will develop gout. Whether your favorite libation is beer or wine may just be one indicator of other lifestyle preferences that also play a role. For example, picture a male beer drinker, then conjure up the image of a male wine drinker. Do you see some significant differences? Is one more likely to be a couch potato? That could be important!

The research study mentioned earlier focused on men, and gout has traditionally been considered a male disease, but researchers have begun to question whether that is true. A high body mass index has been found to increase your risk of developing gout, regardless of your gender. At the November 2005 Annual Scientific Meeting of the

American College of Rheumatology, researchers reported on the results of a study that found women with body mass indexes in the highest category increased their risk of gout sevenfold compared to those in the lowest category. High blood pressure (hypertension) and increased use of diuretics also were strong risk factors for gout. However, women who increased their daily intake of dairy foods strongly decreased their risk of developing gout, just as in the Health Professionals Study of men. This research was presented at the American College of Rheumatology Annual Scientific Meeting.

Good News for Coffee Drinkers

Americans are a nation of coffee drinkers, and we drink an average of two cups each day. You've now read the news about alcohol, meat, and seafood and are probably expecting to hear the same disheartening information about coffee. Surprise! Loving your coffee, even in staggering amounts, doesn't put you at risk for gout.

In 1986, researchers at the Arthritis Research Centre of Canada, the University of British Columbia, Brigham and Women's Hospital, Harvard Medical School, and the Harvard School of Public Health set out to investigate the role of coffee in gout. For this 12-year study, they selected 45,869 men with no history of gout. The men were health professionals, 91 percent were white, and their ages ranged from 40 to 75.

The men reported on their total caffeine and coffee intake, using a food-frequency questionnaire. Researchers broke the long-term coffee drinkers into four groups: those who drank less than one cup per day, one to three cups per day, four to five cups per day, and six or more cups per day. They also considered regular drinkers of decaffeinated coffee, and tea and other caffeinated beverages.

They also evaluated the impact of other risk factors for gout, including body mass index, history of high blood pressure (hypertension), alcohol use, and a diet high in red meat and high-fat dairy foods, along with coffee consumption.

The study's findings, which appeared in the June 2007 issue of *Arthritis & Rheumatism*, indicated that drinking four or more cups of coffee a day dramatically *reduced* men's risk of gout. In fact, the risk of developing gout decreased with increasing coffee consumption. The risk of gout was 40 percent lower for men who drank four to five cups per day and 59 percent lower for men who drank six or more cups per day than for men who never drank coffee.

Decaffeinated coffee also produced positive results, although less so than regular coffee, but tea and total caffeine intake did not have appear to have any effect on the incidence of gout among the participants in the study. It may be that components of coffee apart from caffeine may be at work. Coffee does contain a strong antioxidant, phenol chlorogenic acid.

Signs and Symptoms

Gout generally comes on like the proverbial thief in the night. It's sudden and it's acute. It may hurt to even have the weight of a sheet touch your toe. Intense joint pain, usually affecting the large joint of your big toe, is the giveaway. Gout pain can also occur in your feet, ankles, knees, hands, elbows, and wrists.

The joint or joints affected become swollen, red, and sore. You may also experience a general feeling of malaise, fever, chills, and rapid heartbeat.

If you don't seek treatment, your symptoms will last from five to ten days and then stop, leaving you with some discomfort lasting one to two weeks. This is the pattern of the first attack. Generally, at some point, other attacks will follow.

Diagnosing Gout

Your doctor may suspect gout when you report that you've had one or more episodes of pain at the base of your toes. Ankles and knees are the next most common locations. Gout usually attacks just one joint at a time, unlike rheumatoid arthritis, which attacks multiple joints at the same time.

Your doctor may recommend a blood test to measure the levels of uric acid in your blood. As mentioned, you can have elevated uric acid levels without having gout symptoms and, conversely, you can have gout without having unusually high levels of uric acid.

To make a firm diagnosis, your doctor may draw some fluid from the affected joint (a process known as joint fluid aspiration or arthrocentesis; see Chapter 10) to check for uric acid crystals. Even if you have the classic symptoms of gout, this test can rule out other problems such as pseudogout (discussed later in this chapter), psoriatic arthritis, rheumatoid arthritis, and infection.

X-rays can be helpful for monitoring the effects of chronic gout on your joints and for showing erosions due to crystal deposits or damage to bones caused by inflammation.

Treatment

This is one type of arthritis where prevention is more important than the cure. Keep your fluid intake up, maintain a proper weight, increase your consumption of low-fat dairy products, and eat more complex carbohydrates, such as whole-grain foods.

If you drink alcohol, consider reducing the amount you consume. Cut back on the amount of meat and seafood you eat, and use your prescribed medications to keep your uric acid levels down.

Watch your weight and practice portion control. Losing weight may decrease the uric acid levels in your body. Avoid fad diets or fasting, as these can cause your uric acid levels to fluctuate. Remember to drink plenty of water to help dilute the uric acid in your blood and urine.

Consultation

Watch your consumption of high-protein foods. These include organ meats such as liver, brains, kidneys, and sweet-breads. They are high in purines, and so are anchovies, herring, and mackerel. As purines break down in the body, they produce uric acid.

If you do develop gout in spite of all your precautions, resting and elevating the affected joint can help. Ice packs may help as well, and there are medications available to treat gout. Pain relievers such as acetaminophen can be tried to manage the pain but may not be strong enough. Nonsteroidal anti-inflammatory drugs (NSAIDs) such as indomethacin (Indocin) and naproxen (Naprosyn) can be used to address both pain and inflammation.

Low-dose naproxen is available over the counter as Aleve. Low-dose ibuprofen is available over the counter as Advil. Incocin is available only by prescription. The doses of NSAIDs used to treat acute gout are often quite high and should only be taken under a physician's orders, at least for initial attacks. Once patients are more experienced, some may choose to self-treat.

If your gout is acute, your rheumatologist may prescribe colchicines. These can be taken both orally and intravenously. Corticosteroids, such as prednisone, are used for short-term relief from inflammation. They can be administered orally or injected directly into the inflamed joint.

After the acute phase has subsided, other medications can be taken to lower blood uric acid levels and reduce the risk of recurrent gout attacks over the long term. Probenecid (Benemid) and sulfinpyrazone (Anturane) decrease blood uric acid levels by increasing the excretion of uric acid into the urine. Allopurinol works by blocking the enzyme that converts purines to uric acid and is the drug of choice for people with a history of kidney stones or tophi.

These drugs also reduce your risk of developing kidney stones and kidney disease, and they dissolve crystal deposits.

During the first few months of treatment, you may actually find that you're having more frequent gout attacks and that they're more severe. Patients with gout are usually kept on one or two colchicine pills or one or two NSAID tablets for the first month or two on allopurinol. Even so, some patients may still need to take medication, such as a short course of cortisone, for acute attacks during this interval before the uric acid level has normalized. The first few months of chronic maintenance therapy for gout are a little tricky, so be sure to contact your rheumatologist or primary-care physician if you experience any problems. Within a few months, most people will be free of painful gout episodes as long as they stay on lifetime therapy.

The Outlook

Gout has been called "the scourge of the ages," but researchers today are hard at work to find the cure. Currently, new medications that increase the elimination of uric acid in urine are undergoing clinical trials with patients.

An experimental drug called Y700 is also being tested. Y700 may be able to be used in patients who have kidney disease, because the drug is metabolized by the liver—unlike allopurinol, a commonly used gout medication that is metabolized by the kidneys.

Febuxostat is a new medication that lowers blood uric acid levels. Preliminary studies have shown it to be as effective as allopurinol. It's currently awaiting FDA approval. If it's approved, patients who cannot use allopurinol will have an alternative.

In the meantime, just as with other forms of arthritis, early diagnosis and treatment provide the best outlook.

Pseudogout

Pseudogout is a form of arthritis that shares some common characteristics with gout, but has some important differences. The name itself means "false gout." It's often mistaken for gout and other types of arthritis, but proper and early diagnosis of pseudogout is important, to prevent a severe form of joint degeneration and continued inflammation that can lead to disability.

Consultation _____

Chondrocalcinosis is the name for what's seen on X-rays, while pseudogout is the term for the clinical symptoms of joint pain and swelling that mimic gout.

Pseudogout is caused by deposits of a different kind of crystal, called calcium pyrophosphate, both in and around your joints. It usually affects the knee, but it can also occur in the wrists, shoulders, ankles, elbows, and hands. Pseudogout usually affects just one joint at a time, but it can affect several joints at once. Rarely, you can even have pseudogout at the same time you have gout, in which case two different types of crystals will be found in fluid taken from your joints. That can make you truly miserable.

Who Gets Pseudogout?

Pseudogout equally affects men and women and is more often seen in older people. The average pseudogout patient is over 70 and almost half are 85 or older. It's unusual to find pseudogout in a young person, and if it does develop, it may be a sign of an underlying metabolic disorder. If you have a thyroid condition, kidney failure, or metabolic disorders that involve calcium, phosphate, or iron, you may be at increased risk for developing pseudogout.

Sometimes, people who notice an increase in pain, swelling, and redness around a joint think they're having symptoms of osteoarthritis, when they're actually experiencing an attack of pseudogout. Acute pain, swelling, and redness superimposed upon the chronic low grade aching of osteoarthritis may mean that you have pseudogout as well as OA in that joint.

What Causes Pseudogout?

The American College of Rheumatology reports that pseudogout develops when calcium pyrophosphate crystals accumulate in a joint. First the crystals settle in the cartilage, where they can cause damage. They can also cause an inflammatory response, and this leads to pain and swelling in that joint. We don't know why these crystals form, but we do know that they definitely increase as we age. This fact is leading researchers to investigate a possible connection between the aging process and the development of pseudogout.

The tendency to develop pseudogout runs in families, so there may be a genetic connection at work as well. Other medical conditions such as a severely underactive thyroid (hypothyroidism), excess iron storage (hemochromatosis), low magnesium levels in the blood, an overactive parathyroid gland, and other causes of excessive calcium in the blood (hypercalcemia) can also result in the development of pseudogout.

Injury to your joint can lead to pseudogout, as can either surgery to that joint or surgery done elsewhere on your body. You can't get rid of the crystals, but there are ways to deal with the pain and inflammation of pseudogout.

Signs and Symptoms

Inflammation, swelling, warmth, stiffness, and pain are characteristic symptoms of pseudogout, but they're also symptoms of various other arthritic conditions, including rheumatoid arthritis and osteoarthritis. These symptoms may last for several days or as long as several weeks, and they may leave as quickly as they arrived. Other symptoms include …

- Sudden, intense joint pain.
- A swollen joint that's warm to touch.
- Red or purple skin around the joint.
- Severe tenderness around the joint, so much so that the least amount of pressure or the lightest touch can cause severe pain.

Most of these symptoms will ease within 5 to 12 days, even without treatment. However, sometimes pseudogout can last longer and affect several joints. Over time, pseudogout attacks may occur more often. More joints may be involved and the symptoms may be more severe. These subsequent attacks may last longer than earlier ones.

The pattern is individual. What you experience may very well be quite different from what someone else is experiencing. You may find that you have an attack every few weeks or as infrequently as once a year. The more frequent the attacks, the more joint damage is possible.

Arriving at a Diagnosis

Your rheumatologist will use a needle to withdraw some fluid from the joint that is bothering you and send it to a medical laboratory for crystal identification and other analysis. Even extracting the fluid can relieve your pain, because it removes some of the pressure the fluid has caused.

A diagnosis is made by ruling out other possible causes of joint pain and inflammation. Infection, gout, rheumatoid arthritis, and even an injury are possible other reasons for your pain. X-rays can show if there are crystal deposits in your joint cartilage and if there is damage to the joint.

Treatment

The treatment of pseudogout is similar to the treatment of gout, except that drugs to lower uric acid levels are not prescribed. Decreasing inflammation is the object of treatment for pseudogout. The goal is to slow the progression of joint degeneration.

Nonsteroidal anti-inflammatory drugs (NSAIDs), such as indomethacin (Indocin) and naproxen (Naprosyn), can be prescribed for this purpose. Injection of cortisone into the inflamed joint usually provides prompt relief. In addition, your physician will likely advise you to ice the affected joint and get as much rest as possible. Keeping the joint still can help relieve the pain and swelling. Symptoms may lessen within 24 hours of beginning medication. Colchicine may be prescribed to help prevent future attacks.

In addition to medications, exercise can be helpful. Low-impact exercises (see Chapter 17) can strengthen the muscles around the affected joint and provide relief from pain. Also, regular exercise can help you maintain a proper weight and reduce extra stress on your joints.

Precautions

If you're scheduling elective surgery, be sure to keep well hydrated both before and after your operation. Dehydration has been linked with attacks of pseudogout, especially in the elderly.

Hot and cold compresses can also give relief. Cold packs can reduce pain and swelling, while hot packs help your sore joints relax. You may also find that immobilizing the affected joint for short periods of time is helpful. Your physical therapist may recommend you wear a splint or brace on the joint that's involved.

Prognosis Concerns

The crystal deposits that cause pseudogout can damage your joints. Cysts, bone spurs, and loss of cartilage can develop in the affected joints and, if damage continues, fractures may result. It's important to seek treatment early, since there is currently no treatment available to dissolve the crystal deposits. Once they're there, they remain.

The Least You Need to Know

♦ Gout develops when uric acid crystals deposit in your joints.

♦ Pseudogout develops when calcium pyrophosphate crystals deposit in your joints.

♦ Symptoms of both gout and pseudogout can mimic other diseases, such as a septic joint, osteoarthritis, and rheumatoid arthritis.

♦ Treatment for pseudogout is designed to reduce the pain caused by inflammation but may not slow the progression of joint degeneration.

♦ With proper treatment, the vast majority of gout sufferers should be made painfree.

♦ Both gout and pseudogout can become chronic conditions.

Chapter 8

Related Conditions and Associated Diseases

In This Chapter

- ◆ Autoimmune disease: when your body turns on itself
- ◆ Scleroderma
- ◆ Systemic lupus erythematosus (lupus)
- ◆ Sjögren's syndrome
- ◆ Lyme disease
- ◆ Clearing up confusion between osteoarthritis and osteoporosis

It's entirely possible to have more than one type of arthritis at any given time, and it's also possible for arthritis to develop as part of a related medical condition. In this chapter, we'll discuss some conditions related to arthritis.

Autoimmune Disorders

Your immune system is designed to fight off infection, and it generally does a fine job of recognizing foreign invaders, such as bacteria and viruses, and waging a successful battle against them. Sometimes, however, something goes wrong and the body decides that some of its own tissues are the enemy. It develops *autoantibodies*, which sets the stage for autoimmune disorders to develop.

There are two different kinds of autoimmune disorders. One type is called *systemic*, which means it can affect many organs in your body. The other kind is *localized*, which means just one organ or tissue is directly affected. Scientists don't yet know the exact cause or causes of autoimmune disorders, but some people seem to have an inherited genetic predisposition to develop these diseases, which are then triggered by something in the environment.

def•i•ni•tion

An **autoantibody** is an antibody that turns on itself, attacking the body it's designed to protect.

Scleroderma

Scleroderma, also known as systemic sclerosis, is considered to be a rheumatologic disorder because it affects the body's connective tissues. The word *scleroderma* literally means "hard skin," and this is an accurate description of one of this condition's symptoms. Scleroderma involves overproduction of collagen, the protein that's the building block for bone, cartilage, tendons, and other connective tissues. About 150,000 Americans have scleroderma.

Who Gets Scleroderma?

There are few known risk factors for scleroderma, but a family history appears to be the biggest one. Even among those with a family history, however, fewer than 1 percent will develop scleroderma. Scleroderma usually develops in people between the ages of 35 and 55.

Women are three to eight times more likely than men to develop scleroderma. Children are more likely to have the localized form of scleroderma and adults the systemic form.

What Causes Scleroderma?

The cause or causes aren't yet known, but it's believed that an inherited genetic predisposition to develop scleroderma is triggered by certain environmental factors.

Symptoms of Scleroderma

Symptoms of scleroderma can vary greatly from one person to the next. It can evolve slowly over time, with just a few symptoms, or progress rapidly. The seriousness of this condition depends to a great extent on what parts of the body are affected and how severely they are affected.

Loss of bone in the fingers may not be as severe as that caused by rheumatoid arthritis, but the fingers may shorten over time. When tendons and joints are involved, bending your fingers can become difficult. Muscle weakness can develop, especially around your shoulders and hips.

When your upper digestive tract is involved, you can experience heartburn and difficulty in swallowing, which are symptoms of gastroesophageal reflux disorder (GERD). With lower digestive tract involvement, there can be constipation. If scarring in the lower intestine is severe, watery diarrhea may occur.

> **Consultation**
>
> A mild form of arthritis can develop when scleroderma involves bones, joints, or muscles. This arthritis is usually symmetrical, meaning that the same joints on both sides of the body are affected.

Small white lumps can form beneath the skin—a condition called calcinosis. These lumps sometimes ooze a white substance that looks like toothpaste. Calcinosis can lead to infections.

Scleroderma can cause a loss of small blood vessels at the base of the fingernails in some places and widening of small blood vessels in others. This may be a sign that internal organs have become involved. Over time, the skin can darken overall, with patches of abnormally pale skin. Hair loss can also occur.

Diagnosing Scleroderma

While some patients with scleroderma have specific antibodies, many do not. Your doctor will take your complete medical history and perform a physical examination.

The first step is to determine if your scleroderma is local or systemic, and if it's systemic, determining whether it's a milder form (called limited or CREST) or more widespread (called diffuse).

During the exam, your doctor will check the skin on your fingers and toes for thickened and hardened areas, which is the main clue to detecting scleroderma. He'll also press on the affected tendons and joints to see if there's crackling or a grating sensation, which can indicate changes caused by scleroderma beneath the skin.

Blood tests and other specialized tests can help in arriving at a diagnosis of scleroderma.

Treating Scleroderma

Treatments for specific complications should begin as early as possible, before irreversible hardening of tissues occurs. Rheumatologists and dermatologists can work together to treat this condition. Medications are prescribed to keep blood vessels open and reduce inflammation. These drugs are helpful for improving skin thickness and reducing scarring, even in the lungs. Doctors use other treatments for specific complications, such as proton pump inhibitors for gastrointestinal problems or light treatments for skin thickening.

Prognosis Concerns

As research continues into the causes of scleroderma, scientists are exploring the role certain drugs (some currently being used in cancer treatments) may play in stopping DNA changes from occurring in individuals with scleroderma. Stem cell transplants may also be on the horizon. For more information, visit www.scleroderma.org.

Systemic Lupus Erythematosus

Systemic lupus erythematosus (SLE) is commonly referred to as lupus. It's a chronic inflammatory disease that affects the joints, kidneys, lungs, nervous system, skin, or other organs of the body. Lupus can be difficult to diagnose, since its symptoms mimic those of many other medical conditions.

The American College of Rheumatology notes that lupus ranges from mild to severe, typically involving alternating periods of activity and remission. Lupus is a very serious disease, but therapy can increase life expectancy and significantly improve quality of life.

Who Gets Lupus?

Lupus typically develops in people in their 20s and 30s. It occurs 10 times more often in women than in men, is three times more common in African American women than in Caucasian women, and is also more common in women of Hispanic, Asian, and Native American descent. It's difficult to estimate how many people in the United States have lupus because symptoms vary so widely and the onset of the disease is often difficult to determine.

What Causes Lupus?

The National Institutes of Health (NIH) reports that lupus likely results from a combination of genetic, environmental, and possibly hormonal factors. Lupus has been found to run in families, but it is still rare for more than one individual in a family to have lupus.

Symptoms of Lupus

Symptoms can develop gradually and the pattern can vary from person to person. This can make diagnosing lupus difficult. The most common symptoms include skin rashes and arthritis, often accompanied by fatigue and fever. Other symptoms include …

- Weight loss.
- A butterfly-shaped rash over the cheeks or other rashes in areas exposed to the sun.
- Sores in the mouth or nose, lasting for more than a month.
- Loss of hair, sometimes in spots or around the hairline.
- Seizures and strokes.
- Blood clots.
- Miscarriages.
- Chest pain when taking deep breaths.
- Heartburn.
- Abdominal pain.
- Poor circulation to the fingers and toes.

According to the National Institute of Arthritis and Musculoskeletal and Skin Diseases, new symptoms may continue to appear for years after the disease's first appearance. Different symptoms may arise at different times. In some lupus sufferers, only the skin or joints are affected. Others experience symptoms in many parts of the body.

Diagnosing Lupus

It may take months or even years to diagnose this complex disease accurately, and arriving at a correct diagnosis is truly a team effort. According to the National Institute of Arthritis and Musculoskeletal and Skin Diseases, you can expect your physician to take a complete medical history, conduct a physical examination, and order laboratory tests (including blood work and urinalysis). X-rays and other imaging tests may be used to see affected organs. Skin and kidney biopsies can help confirm the diagnosis.

> ### Straight Talk
>
> It took months to get a diagnosis of lupus. My doctor thought I was too old for lupus and was treating me for rheumatoid arthritis. The treatment is very similar, but at least I know what I have now.
>
> —Linda, age 62

Blood tests will reveal if the antinuclear antibody (ANA) is present. This antibody is present in virtually everyone with lupus. However, it's important to know that many more people have a "false positive" ANA. More than 95 percent of all positive ANAs occur in people who do not have lupus, including many who are completely healthy.

Treating Lupus

Treating lupus is a team effort. You and your rheumatologist will be the primary team members, but there's a whole cadre of health-care professionals ready to help you.

A hematologist is a doctor specializing in blood disorders. People with lupus may develop anemia, leukopenia (a decreased number of white blood cells), or thrombocytopenia (a decrease in the number of platelets, which assist in clotting). Some people with lupus may have an increased risk of blood clots.

A nephrologist is a doctor specializing in treating kidney disease. When lupus involves your kidneys, intensive and aggressive treatment is necessary to prevent permanent loss of kidney function.

A neurologist is a doctor specializing in disorders of the nervous system. Lupus can affect the brain and central nervous system, causing headaches, dizziness, memory problems, vision problems, stroke, seizures, or behavioral changes.

A cardiologist is a doctor specializing in diseases involving the heart. In some people with lupus, inflammation can occur in the heart itself (myocarditis and endocarditis) or the membrane that surrounds it (pericarditis), causing chest pain or other symptoms. Lupus can also increase the risk of atherosclerosis (hardening of the arteries).

A cardiopulmonary specialist treats diseases involving the lungs as well as the heart. Some people with lupus develop pleuritis, an inflammation of the lining of the chest cavity that causes chest pain, particularly with breathing. Pneumonia can be a concern if your lungs are involved, so it's important to treat all respiratory infections promptly.

Consultation

You can do your part to prevent complications by reducing other risk factors for heart disease. If you smoke, quit. If you have high blood pressure, take medication to control it. If your cholesterol is high, make healthy dietary changes, exercise, and take prescribed medication, if necessary.

If muscle or joint pain, a rash, or fatigue are the extent of your lupus symptoms, your rheumatologist may prescribe a nonsteroidal anti-inflammatory drug (NSAID), such as ibuprofen (Motrin, Advil) or naproxen (Naprosyn). Hydroxychloroquine (Plaquenil), originally an antimalarial medication, may also be prescribed. Low doses of prednisone may also be given.

More serious or life-threatening symptoms, such as kidney inflammation, heart or lung involvement, or central nervous system involvement, necessitate more aggressive treatment. In these circumstances, your rheumatologist may prescribe high-dose corticosteroids such as prednisone (Deltasone) and other immunosuppressive drugs such as azathioprine (Imuran), cyclophosphamide (Cytoxan), or cyclosporine (Neoral, Sandimmune). Recently, mycophenolate mofetil (CellCept) has been used to treat severe lupus-related kidney disease.

Precautions

According to the American College of Rheumatology, if you have lupus, you should limit your exposure to the sun. Ultraviolet rays can cause a skin rash to flare, possibly even triggering a more serious flare in the disease itself. Be sure to wear protective clothing and use sunscreen when outdoors.

Sometimes several medications are combined to get the best results. For a more in-depth look at medications used to treat lupus and other rheumatologic conditions, see Chapter 9.

Pregnancy and Lupus

Pregnancy with lupus is considered high risk. Women with lupus have higher rates of miscarriage and premature births than the general population. If you are considering becoming pregnant, pregnancy counseling and planning can increase your chances of safely carrying your baby to term. It's recommended that you have no symptoms of active lupus and be on a stable medication for at least six months prior to becoming pregnant.

Prognosis Concerns

A major funding agent for lupus research is the National Institute of Arthritis and Musculoskeletal and Skin Diseases (NIAMS), a component of the National Institutes of Health (NIH). Researchers at the NIAMS on-campus program in Bethesda, Maryland, are evaluating patients with lupus and their relatives to discover more about how lupus develops and changes over time.

Additional projects include studying the genetic factors that increase a person's risk of developing lupus, specialized centers devoted specifically to lupus research, and lupus registries that gather medical information, as well as blood and tissue samples, from patients and their relatives. These samples are then made available to researchers.

Other areas of research include investigations into why more women than men develop lupus. Scientists suspect that hormones may play a role in the development and the course of lupus. A current study funded by the NIH is focusing on the safety and effectiveness of oral contraceptives (birth control pills) and hormone replacement therapy in women with lupus. Previous studies have shown that low-dose birth control pills are probably safe if you have mild lupus. For more information, check out the Lupus Foundation of America at www.lupus.org.

Consultation

People with lupus may have a genetic defect that prevents the body from naturally eliminating cells that have reached the end of their lives, a process called apoptosis or "programmed cell death." If these cells remain in the body, they can interfere with other cells and may play a role in disease development.

Sjögren's Syndrome

Sjögren's syndrome is an autoimmune disease. In Sjogren's, the immune system attacks the body's moisture-producing glands. About half the time, Sjögren's syndrome occurs alone, a condition called primary Sjögren's. The rest of the time, it occurs with another connective tissue disease, such as rheumatoid arthritis, lupus, scleroderma, or polymyositis/dermatomyositis. This is referred to as secondary Sjögren's.

Who Gets Sjögren's Syndrome?

Sjögren's syndrome is one of the most common autoimmune disorders, affecting as many as 4,000,000 Americans. Nine out of ten individuals with Sjögren's syndrome are women. The average age of onset is the late 40s, although Sjögren's occurs in all age groups in both women and men.

What Causes Sjögren's Syndrome?

The exact cause of Sjögren's syndrome is not yet known, but scientists believe genetic factors are significantly responsible, since it's sometimes found in more than one family member. Several different genes appear to be involved. It is also found more commonly in families that have members with other autoimmune illnesses, such as lupus.

To add another layer to the genetic mystery, one gene predisposes Caucasians to Sjögren's, but other genes are linked to Sjögren's in individuals of Japanese, Chinese, or African American ancestry. But even if you have these genes, it doesn't mean you will develop Sjögren's. There needs to be some sort of trigger, possibly something in the environment, such as a viral infection, that activates the immune system.

Symptoms of Sjögren's Syndrome

The classic symptoms are dry eyes and dry mouth. Sjögren's may also involve other organs, affecting the kidneys, gastrointestinal tract, blood vessels, lungs, liver, pancreas, and central nervous system. Other symptoms include extreme fatigue and joint pain. Some people experience mild symptoms, while others can become disabled. The symptoms can get worse, level off, or even go into remission.

Diagnosing Sjögren's Syndrome

The average time from onset of symptoms to diagnosis is more than six years. There are several reasons why. First of all, symptoms can be similar to those of lupus, rheumatoid arthritis, fibromyalgia, chronic fatigue syndrome, and multiple sclerosis. Additionally, having dry eyes or a dry mouth can be caused by side effects of certain medications, and this can make the diagnosis more difficult.

Also, not all symptoms are always present at the same time. If Sjögren's involves more than one body system, you may find yourself being treated by two different health professionals, such as your dentist and your primary-care physician, who don't know that they're dealing with a larger picture.

Once your physician has determined that Sjögren's syndrome may be responsible for your symptoms, blood tests can help make a definitive diagnosis. Once the diagnosis has been made, you may be referred to an ophthalmologist and an oral pathologist or dentist for additional tests and procedures.

Precautions _____

> In one study reported in 2001, the incidence of lymphoma (cancer of the lymph glands) was found to be 44 times higher in people with Sjögren's syndrome than in the general population. It's important to be in close communication with your rheumatologist if you develop symptoms such as rapidly enlarging lymph nodes or a large, hard parotid gland.

Many symptoms of Sjögren's syndrome can be treated with over-the-counter medications, such as preservative-free artificial tears, artificial salivas, saline nasal sprays, and vaginal lubricants. For more serious problems, a variety of prescription medications can be added. In addition, a humidifier and protective eyewear, such as goggles, can be helpful. The Sjögren's Syndrome Foundation can provide you with a list of products to make your life easier and has a newsletter that gives suggestions and tips for daily living.

Prognosis Concerns

Sjögren's syndrome is a potentially serious but generally not fatal condition if complications are diagnosed and treated early. The Sjögren's Syndrome Foundation has good information on current research into the causes and treatments for this condition. Visit www.sjogrens.org for more information.

Lyme Disease

Lyme disease gets its name from Lyme, Connecticut, the site where it was discovered in 1975. A number of children in Lyme and the surrounding area developed symptoms of juvenile arthritis (JA), which raised some questions. Eventually it was learned that most of the children lived near wooded areas and, though not all of them could remember having been bitten by a tick, the onset of their symptoms seemed to coincide with the height of the summer tick season. Since that time, Lyme disease has spread across most of the United States, and cases have also been reported in Europe, Asia, and South America.

What Causes Lyme Disease?

Deer ticks infected with a spirochete (a type of organism smaller than a bacterium but bigger than a virus), which was later named *Borrelia burgdorferi*, turned out to be the cause. The majority of these ticks have been found in New York, Connecticut, New Jersey, Minnesota, and Wisconsin.

Deer aren't the only animals that harbor these ticks. White-footed field mice, raccoons, opossums, skunks, weasels, foxes, shrews, moles, chipmunks, squirrels, and horses are also hosts.

If you are pregnant, be especially careful to avoid ticks in areas where Lyme disease is prevalent. A prenatal infection can increase your risk of miscarriage, and the infection can be transferred to your unborn child.

Consultation

Deer populations have been increasing in the Northeast and people have been moving into rural areas. The combination has resulted in people coming in closer contact with everything that lives in the woods—ticks are no exception.

Symptoms of Lyme Disease

Flu-like symptoms can develop in the early stages of Lyme disease. These include fever and chills, headache, muscle and joint pain, and stiff neck, swollen lymph glands, and a general sense of malaise. Later, nerve, heart, and brain problems can occur, along with arthritis, often in the knees.

Lyme disease imitates a variety of illnesses and its severity can vary from person to person. If you have been bitten by a tick and live in an area known to have Lyme disease, see your doctor right away so that a proper diagnosis can be made and treatment started.

A bulls-eye rash at the initial bite site is a characteristic early symptom, appearing within a week or so of a person's being bitten, although not every person who has been bitten develops a rash. The rash is called erythema migrans. As the infection spreads, several rashes can appear at different sites on the body.

Lyme disease can affect many different organs in your body, causing respiratory problems, nervous system problems, and joint problems.

Diagnosing Lyme Disease

Lyme disease can be difficult to diagnose because many of its symptoms mimic those of other conditions and because many people don't remember having been bitten. In about one fourth of people infected, there is no rash, so if the rash isn't present, your doctor may order blood tests to try to identify the cause.

Lyme antibody tests can indicate either recent or more remote exposure to the Lyme organism. Over the years since the original discovery of Lyme disease, testing has improved to the point that there are now more accurate laboratory tests with fewer false negative and false positive results. If you're experiencing nervous system symptoms, your doctor may order a spinal tap, which is a procedure in which spinal fluid is removed from the spinal canal and sent to a laboratory for examination. This will determine if you have antibodies fighting the spirochete. It will also detect any inflammation in your brain or spinal cord.

Treating and Preventing Lyme Disease

In its early stages, Lyme disease can be effectively treated with antibiotics. In general, the sooner such therapy is begun, the quicker and more complete the recovery.

Prevention is important, and there are many steps you can take to decrease your risk of being bitten by a tick. Most people become infected during the late spring, summer, and early fall when immature ticks have hatched and are out and about. Except in warm climates, few people are bitten by deer ticks during winter months. Deer ticks are most often found in wooded areas and nearby grasslands, and they are especially common where the two areas merge, including neighborhood yards where deer occasionally roam. Ticks do not survive long on sunny lawns, as they dry out quickly and die.

Consultation

There was a vaccine (LYMErix) available for Lyme disease, but poor sales caused the makers to remove it from the market.

To reduce your chances of getting bitten by a tick, follow these tips:

♦ Wear long sleeves and tightly woven clothing that is light in color when walking in wooded areas, so the ticks can be seen more easily if you happen to collect any.

♦ Tuck your shirt into your pants and tuck your pants into your socks or boots.

♦ Walk in the center of trails through the woods to avoid picking up ticks from overhanging grass and brush.

♦ Keep grass mowed as short as possible.

♦ Apply tick repellents containing DEET to your clothing, shoes, and socks before going out. Another tick repellent, called permethrin, is designed to be placed on the clothing and can be used alone or in combination with DEET.

♦ Check yourself, your family, and your pets routinely for ticks, especially after being outdoors.

♦ Shower and shampoo your hair if you think you may have been exposed to ticks.

♦ Check your clothes for ticks and wash them immediately in order to remove any ticks.

In spite of all these precautions, if you are still bitten, you have time. If the tick has just latched on, you can remove it safely. The tick will not transmit the bacterium until it has finished its meal of your blood.

To remove a tick that has attached itself to your skin, tug gently but firmly with blunt tweezers near the head of the tick until it releases its hold. Keep your handling of the tick to a minimum to lessen your chance of coming in contact with the bacterium. Try not to crush the tick's body or to touch the tick with bare fingers. When you have removed the tick, swab the bite area thoroughly with an antiseptic to prevent infection. Removing an infected tick within 24 hours greatly reduces the chance of developing Lyme disease.

Precautions

Do not use kerosene, Vaseline, a lit match, or a cigarette butt to remove the tick. Any of these methods can cause the tick's head to remain in your skin and transmit the bacterium.

Prognosis Concerns

Most people who contract Lyme disease recover completely after a course of antibiotics. Some people may have persistent symptoms or symptoms that recur, making further antibiotic treatment necessary. If left untreated, Lyme disease can cause permanent damage to the heart, nervous system, and joints.

Having had Lyme disease once doesn't give you immunity, so you can get re-infected if you are bitten by another tick that carries the bacterium. Prevention remains the best option.

An Important Word About Osteoporosis

The similarity between the names *osteoarthritis* and *osteoporosis* has caused much confusion among the general public about these very different medical conditions. In an effort to clear up this confusion, the National Osteoporosis Foundation (NOF) has issued an urgent public health advisory concerning these diseases. The pamphlet, titled "What People with Arthritis Need to Know About Osteoporosis," is available from the National Osteoporosis Foundation (www.nofstore.org/Merchant2/merchant. mvc?Screen=PROD&Product_Code=B116A&Category_Code=).

The NOF is particularly concerned that many women may not realize that, unlike arthritis, osteoporosis is a symptomless, painless disease until a fracture occurs. The advisory warns women that waiting for the onset of symptoms before being evaluated for their risk of osteoporosis may have dangerous consequences.

The NOF is particularly concerned that the confusion relating to osteoporosis and osteoarthritis may be an important reason why people may fail to take needed and effective action to prevent and treat osteoporosis. For example …

- Recent surveys found that six in ten people think that osteoporosis has warning signs or symptoms when it actually has no signs or symptoms until a bone fracture occurs.

- One in two women surveyed incorrectly believe that the treatment of osteoporosis and arthritis are similar.

- Forty-two percent of women mistakenly believe that osteoporosis and arthritis are always related disorders.

Osteoporosis causes loss of bone tissue, leading to increased risk of fractures. It can lead to permanent disability, but it's a silent disease—the first symptom is usually a fracture.

The bottom line is that osteoarthritis is a form of arthritis—the most common form. Osteoporosis is *not* a form of arthritis. It is an entirely different medical condition. It's possible to have both arthritis and osteoporosis at the same time. Studies have found that people with osteoarthritis are less likely to develop osteoporosis, but people with rheumatoid arthritis are more likely to develop osteoporosis. It's a major health threat for 44 million Americans, 68 percent of whom are women.

The Least You Need to Know

- Autoimmune disease can affect just one organ or body tissue, or it can involve many organ systems.

- Scleroderma is an autoimmune disease that causes hardening of the skin.

- Lupus is a chronic inflammatory disease that can affect the joints, along with many of the body's organs.

- Sjögren's syndrome is an autoimmune disease that attacks the body's moisture-producing glands.

- Lyme disease results from a tick bite, so take preventive measures when out-doors.

- Osteoarthritis and osteoporosis may sound alike, but they're two very different conditions.

Part 3

The Path to Treatment

The process of moving from accurate diagnosis to effective treatment takes time, and when you're in pain, the wait can seem interminable. There's a great deal that goes on during this critical period, and understanding just what's involved can help you become an active participant rather than a passive observer. In Part 3, you'll take a guided journey along the path from diagnosis to treatment.

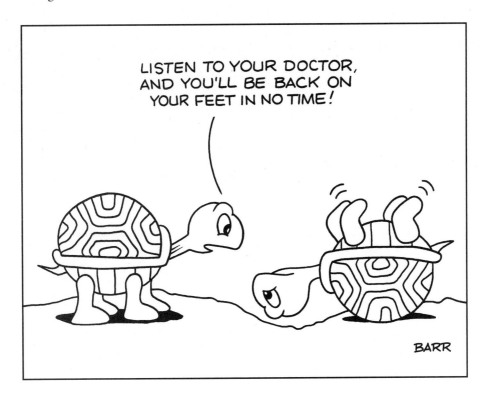

Arthritis Medications

In This Chapter

- The right medication for your type of arthritis
- How your medications work
- Guarding against side effects
- Buying your medications with confidence

Both prescription and over-the-counter medications are available to help you manage your arthritis symptoms. Some of these medications target pain, while others focus on reducing inflammation or preventing the progression of certain types of arthritis. In this chapter, you'll learn what those drugs are, how they work, and what kind of relief you can expect from them.

Pain Relievers

Your first concern with arthritis is addressing your pain. Medications that do this are called analgesics, and they relieve pain by blocking the brain's reception of pain signals or by changing the way the brain interprets these signals. Analgesics can be broken into two categories: the non-narcotics and the *narcotics*.

def•i•ni•tion

A **narcotic** is a drug that reduces pain, alters mood or behavior, and usually induces sleep or stupor. Narcotics are stronger pain relievers than analgesics but also have the potential to be addictive.

Aspirin and certain other pain relievers can also be used to treat inflammation. These drugs are called nonsteroidal anti-inflammatory drugs (NSAIDs) and you'll read more about them shortly.

Non-Narcotic Pain Relievers

Acetaminophen (Tylenol) is an example of a non-narcotic analgesic. It does not have anti-inflammatory properties. The most commonly used over-the-counter medication for mild to moderate pain relief, it's generally effective for aches and pains associated with mild arthritis.

The usual recommended dose of acetaminophen extra-strength tablets is 500 mg to 1000 mg every four to six hours as needed, not to exceed a maximum of 4000 mg per day. The usual recommended dose of acetaminophen arthritis-strength 650mg tablets is 1300 mg every eight hours, up to a maximum daily dose of 3990 mg.

Narcotic Pain Relievers

Narcotics are strong painkillers usually prescribed to address acute intense pain. They may also be effective in treating chronic pain. They work by blocking pain signals traveling to the brain. They do not relieve inflammation.

Precautions

Acetaminophen is an ingredient in many over-the-counter cold and flu medications. If you are already taking acetaminophen for your arthritis pain, check with your physician or pharmacist before using any of these preparations in order to avoid an overdose.

Common side effects of narcotics use include constipation, dry mouth, difficulty with urination, drowsiness, contraction of the pupils (called miosis), and a drop in blood pressure with sudden change to a standing position (called orthostatic hypotension). If you are already taking medications that may cause drowsiness, check with your physician before beginning a course of narcotic treatment.

Narcotics have other less common, serious side effects. These include confusion and hallucinations, delirium, itching and hives, hypothermia, and a slow heart rate (called bradycardia) or a rapid heart rate (called tachycardia). There may be an increase in pressure within the brain cavity (intracranial pressure), spasms of the bile duct or the urethra, muscle rigidity, and flushing. Respiratory depression and death may occur with an overdose.

There are numerous narcotic drugs:

- Tylenol with codeine (acetaminophen with codeine)

- Morphine (MS Contin)

- Darvocet (propoxyphene with acetaminophen)

- Darvon (propoxyphene)

- Duragesic (fentanyl patch)

- Palladone, Dilaudid (hydromorphone)

- OxyContin, Roxicodone (oxycodone)

- Percodan (oxycodone with aspirin)

- Talwin NX (pentazocine with naloxone)

- Lorcet, Lortab, Vicodin (hydrocodone with acetaminophen)

- Percocet (oxycodone with acetaminophen)

Extended use of narcotics comes with a risk of dependency, which means your body requires more and more of the drug in order to achieve the desired effect. You may experience symptoms of drug withdrawal if you suddenly discontinue your narcotic prescription without a gradual tapering off. To prevent this, your physician will generally prescribe the lowest effective dose for the shortest time period necessary to treat your symptoms.

Consultation

Ultram (tramadol) and Ultracet (tramadol with acetaminophen), which also belong to the narcotic class of medications, have less potential for addiction and withdrawal symptoms.

Attacking Inflammation

One class of drugs used to treat inflammation is called nonsteroidal anti-inflammatory drugs. As you can tell by the name, these drugs do not contain steroids. These drugs are commonly called NSAIDs (pronounced *N-sayds*).

NSAIDs are included in many cold and allergy medications. They help relieve mild to moderate joint pain, fever, stiffness, and swelling. NSAIDs work by blocking specific enzymes and reducing levels of chemicals called *prostaglandins*.

def•i•ni•tion

Prostaglandins are produced by the body's cells and are found in nearly all of the body's tissues and organs. They work hard! They help send pain messages to the brain and also promote inflammation and fever, support the function of platelets necessary for blood to clot, and protect the stomach from acid damage.

How NSAIDs Work

To understand how NSAIDs work, you first need to get acquainted with two important prostaglandins, known as COX-1 and COX-2. COX-1 is the good guy, protecting your stomach and producing platelets. COX-2 is the bad guy, promoting inflammation.

NSAIDs are COX-1 and COX-2 inhibitors; they reduce the production of prostaglandins. NSAIDs vary in strength, in duration of effectiveness, and in the way they are eliminated from the body. The stronger the NSAID, the greater the possibility of side effects. Side effects of NSAIDs include stomach ulcers and bleeding.

An NSAID that is a selective COX inhibitor targets primarily COX-2. For example, celecoxib (Celebrex) is a COX-2 inhibitor, and has little effect on COX-1. It tends to cause less bleeding and fewer stomach ulcers than other NSAIDs but may carry an added risk for coronary artery disease. Numerous NSAIDs are commonly prescribed:

- Aspirin
- Salsalate (Amigesic)
- Diflunisal (Dolobid)
- Ibuprofen (Motrin, Advil, Nuprin)
- Ketoprofen (Orudis)

- Nabumetone (Relafen)

- Piroxicam (Feldene)

- Naproxen (Aleve, Naprosyn)

- Diclofenac (Voltaren)

- Indomethacin (Indocin)

- Sulindac (Clinoril)

- Tolmetin (Tolectin)

- Etodolac (Lodine)

- Ketorolac (Toradol)

- Oxaprozin (Daypro)

- Celecoxib (Celebrex)

Doubling Up on NSAIDs

Over-the-counter purchase of NSAIDs has become commonplace, and this easy access can lead to a nonchalant attitude toward them. This can be dangerous. If your physician prescribes an NSAID for the same or a different condition, twice as much medication is entering your body and the potential for serious side effects is increased. So it's important to tell all your doctors what over-the-counter medications you are taking.

Side Effects

The most common side effects of NSAIDs are nausea, vomiting, diarrhea, or constipation. You may notice a decrease in appetite and may develop a rash, dizziness, headache, or drowsiness. Fluid retention (edema) is also a possible side effect.

The most serious side effects are kidney or liver failure, elevated blood pressure, stomach ulcers, and risk of prolonged bleeding. Your risk of side effects increases with long-term use of NSAIDs.

Precautions

It is possible to be allergic to one or more of the NSAIDs. If you have asthma, be aware of your increased risk of a severe allergic reaction. People who find that aspirin causes wheezing should avoid all NSAIDs.

Subdividing NSAIDs

You're probably familiar with the use of aspirin as a blood thinner to prevent heart attacks. Aspirin's ability to keep blood from clotting is not always a good thing, however, as it can increase your risk of bleeding. That's why you're told to discontinue your use of aspirin and other NSAIDS a couple of weeks before having surgery.

Aspirin is an NSAID and it's also a salicylate; in fact, its name tells you so (acetylsalicylic acid or ASA). Other NSAIDs do not have as strong an anticlotting effect and are less likely to cause bleeding or bleeding ulcers at prescribed doses. These nonacetylated compounds include salsalate (Disalcid), choline magnesium trisalicylate (Trilisate), and magnesium salicylate.

If you find that one of the narcotics or a NSAID is not effective in relieving your pain, your physician may consider an NSAID-narcotic combination to get better results.

Steroids

Steroids are synthetic drugs related to cortisol, a naturally occurring hormone that controls many important body functions. This class of drugs relieves pain as a secondary function by reducing swelling and inflammation. You will hear your physician refer to them as corticosteroids or glucocorticoids.

Corticosteroids are useful in treating several rheumatic conditions:

- Bursitis
- Dermatomyositis
- Giant cell arteritis
- Gout
- Osteoarthritis (as local injections, not orally)
- Polymyalgia rheumatica
- Polymyositis
- Pseudogout
- Rheumatoid arthritis
- Systemic lupus erythematosus (lupus)
- Tendinitis (as local injections, not orally)
- Vasculitis

Because of the potential for side effects, steroids are usually prescribed in low doses for the shortest possible period of time. Cortisone, prednisone, and methylprednisolone are common corticosteroids.

These medications are often taken in pill form, but they may also be injected directly into the joint or bursa to treat osteoarthritis and bursitis. To treat other conditions, they may be injected into a muscle or a vein. Too frequent injections, however, can result in serious side effects.

In some cases where high doses of steroids are required—for example, when lupus has involved the kidneys, nervous system, or brain—"pulse" corticosteroids are injected directly into the vein for no more than three consecutive days. This procedure is usually performed by a rheumatologist or other physician in a hospital, due to the potential for serious side effects.

Consultation

Corticosteroids prescribed to treat arthritis are not the same as the performance-enhancement drugs used by athletes. Those drugs are anabolic steroids.

Steroids are also available in lotion or cream form to treat skin conditions, such as psoriasis, associated with certain kinds of arthritis. Eyedrops containing corticosteroids can be used to treat certain eye conditions associated with arthritis. Nasal sprays are used to treat allergies. Steroids in the form of creams, eyedrops, sprays, and injections into joints or bursa generally cause fewer side effects in other parts of the body than do pills.

Prednisone

Prednisone is a corticosteroid taken by mouth to treat the inflammatory types of arthritis, such as rheumatoid arthritis (RA). Recent studies have shown it may not only decrease joint swelling and pain, but may also slow the progression of joint damage in early RA. Corticosteroids such as prednisone or prednisolone may be prescribed early on to control inflammation until other disease-modifying drugs (covered in the next section) have time to take effect.

Prednisone comes with a laundry list of potential side effects, ranging from mild to severe:

◆ Weight gain, either water retention or true weight gain due to increased appetite

◆ Mood swings, either positive or negative

- Weakness in the muscles of arms or legs (myopathy)

- Blurred vision due to elevated blood sugar, elevated pressure in the eye (glaucoma), or cataracts

- Round face and increased fat deposits in the upper back and abdomen

- Slowed growth rate in children and adolescents

- Infections due to suppression of the immune system

- High blood pressure, elevated blood sugar, and stomach irritation or stomach ulcers (especially when in combination with aspirin or NSAIDs)

- Acne, slow healing of cuts and wounds, easy bruising, and red or purple stretch marks

- Thinning hair or excessive hair growth

- Osteoporosis resulting in hip or spinal fractures

- Osteonecrosis, a serious and painful bone condition occurring most often in the hip or shoulder when the bone is deprived of circulation

The seriousness of side effects tends to be in proportion to the steroid dosage and length of treatment. Many people tolerate low-dose steroids for long periods of time with minimal, if any, side effects.

Prednisone During Pregnancy

Prednisone can be used safely during pregnancy, but both your ob-gyn and your rheumatologist need to be involved in the decision to prescribe it and work together to provide you with optimum benefits and the fewest complications. Many times a perinatologist (a specialist in "high risk" obstetrics) is also called in. If you wish to breast feed, be aware that your breast milk will contain prednisone. Discuss this issue with your physician to develop an appropriate course of action.

Tapering Off Prednisone

If treatment with steroids brings your arthritis symptoms under better control, it is important to reduce your dosage over a period of time. *Tapering off steroids should always be done with the knowledge and direction of your physician.* Abruptly stopping steroid use can be dangerous. You may experience withdrawal symptoms unless you gradually decrease your dosage. These symptoms can include muscle, bone, and joint aches; fever; weight loss; headache; and nausea. These symptoms are generally short-lived, lasting up to two weeks.

 Precautions

If you develop symptoms during the tapering withdrawal period, be sure to check with your doctor to determine whether these are due to withdrawal from cortico-steroids or due to a flare.

Alternate-Day Schedule

If your doctor has prescribed high-dose steroids for a long period of time, she may suggest that you take a higher dose of your corticosteroid one day and a lower dose or no dose the following day. The goal is to keep your symptoms under control while reducing the potential for side effects.

Lag Time

After you have discontinued corticosteroids, it takes some time for your body to resume its normal production of those hormones. This can be important if you have surgery scheduled. Your doctor may prescribe a "boost" of corticosteroids prior to sur-gery to ensure appropriate levels.

Adding Another Layer of Treatment

A class of drugs that not only relieves pain and reduces inflammation, but that actually slows down or stops the progression of joint damage is called disease-modifying anti-rheumatic drugs (DMARDs).

DMARDs are used to treat rheumatoid arthritis (RA), ankylosing spondylitis, and psoriatic arthritis. The drugs may take several weeks or months to become effective. DMARDs include methotrexate (Rheumatrex), hydroxychloroquine (Plaquenil), sul-fasalazine (Azulfidine), and leflunomide (Arava).

Methotrexate

Methotrexate (Rheumatrex, Trexall) is often the first line of DMARD treatment for rheumatoid arthritis. It's frequently prescribed along with other medications. It's given as a single dose once a week either orally or by injection and works to relieve pain and stiffness and helps combat fatigue.

Methotrexate directly targets the immune system to fight inflammation and to prevent joint damage. It's generally prescribed for long-term use. When discontinued, symptoms often recur. While serious side effects are uncommon at the doses of methotrexate used to treat RA, regular laboratory testing is required. Women who are planning on becoming pregnant should be off methotrexate for at least two to three months before trying to conceive.

Arava

Arava works to reduce inflammation associated with RA. Arava is administered as a pill with a dose of 10 or 20 mg daily. A loading dose of 100 mg daily for two or three days followed by the 10 or 20 mg daily dose is the usual course.

Possible side effects include rash, reversible hair loss, irritation of the liver, nausea, diarrhea, and abdominal pain. Periodic blood tests are needed to check liver function. Arava is not recommended for people with liver disease; women who are nursing, pregnant, or may become pregnant; or people with an immune deficiency or disorder.

Consultation

Sometimes a drug developed to treat one condition is found to also have benefit in treating an unrelated condition. Plaquenil was originally used as an antimalarial drug, but people taking it also reported improvement in their arthritis symptoms. Chemotherapy medications such as methotrexate, Cytoxan, and Imuran were also found to be helpful in treating RA.

Plaquenil

Plaquenil works on the immune system and is often used as the initial DMARD in patients with mild RA. Plaquenil is also used to treat the facial rash symptomatic of lupus. It can be used in combination with steroid treatment to reduce the amount of steroid required. Plaquenil is taken orally. Side effects are rare, but may include skin rash, low white blood cell count, blood or protein in the urine, and nausea. High doses over years of treatment may very rarely cause injury to the back of the eye, so regular monitoring by an ophthalmologist is indicated.

Gold

Gold salts are rarely prescribed now, but they were used to treat RA from the 1920s until the mid-1980s. Gold decreases joint inflammation and is administered either orally or by injection into the muscle—the more effective method. Side effects can include rash, anemia, low white blood cell count, and liver and kidney problems.

Cyclosporine

Cyclosporine (Neoral) was initially a drug given to prevent rejection of transplanted organs. Because it's designed to keep the immune system from turning on the body, it can also be useful in treating joint inflammation associated with rheumatoid arthritis. Its side effects include nausea, diarrhea, heartburn, kidney problems, high blood pressure, and headache. Other DMARDs without these potential side effects tend to be prescribed more often.

Azulfidine

Another DMARD, Azulfidine, is used to treat rheumatoid arthritis, the arthritis associated with ankylosing spondylitis and IBD. It can be used alone or in combination with other drugs.

The Biologics

The biologics are an exciting new development in the treatment of severe arthritis. Like laser-guided cruise missiles, these medications target very specific parts of the immune system. They are called biologic response modifiers (BRMs) or biologics and are a newer class of DMARDs.

If you have severe rheumatoid, ankylosing spondylitis, or psoriatic arthritis, biologics can often give you dramatic improvement. This is true even with very severe disease that has been resistant to methotrexate and other traditional DMARDs. Results are seen almost always within three months of starting treatment.

The biologics are substances that occur naturally in the human body in small amounts. Biologics in use include Enbrel (etanercept), Humira (adalimumab), Kineret (anakinra), Orencia (abatacept), Rituxan (rituximab), and Remicade (infliximab). Both DMARDs and biologics are designed to promote remission.

Side Effects

Side effects are usually short term and disappear after the course of treatment. They can include flu-like symptoms of chills, fever, muscle aches, weakness, nausea, vomiting, diarrhea, and loss of appetite. Other side effects include a rash and a tendency to bruise or bleed easily.

Biologics are not yet available in oral form and must be administered by injection or infusion. Mild skin reactions (minor swelling, itching, and redness) at the site of injection are a common side effect. Some patients report headaches during intravenous infusion. Increased susceptibility to infection is another possible side effect.

How They Work

Since the biologics work by depressing certain immune system functions, it is essential to monitor your health carefully when taking these drugs. If you have another medical condition, such as diabetes, that may make you prone to infection or if you have a history of tuberculosis, consult your rheumatologist prior to beginning treatment with biologics. If you develop an infection that requires an antibiotic while taking these drugs, you may need to postpone your injections until you have finished your antibiotics and your infection has cleared up.

Biologics work quickly to reduce inflammation, often within two weeks of beginning a course of treatment. This is in contrast to DMARDs, which may take one to six months to achieve the same result. Some biologics are used in combination with DMARDs, particularly methotrexate, to achieve maximum effectiveness.

Research into new biologics is continuing and hopefully will result in treatment options for the 25 percent of rheumatoid arthritis patients who do not respond to the currently available biologics.

Biologic therapy is expensive, with annual costs ranging from $17,000 to $25,000 or more, depending on the drug. The cost reflects the long and involved path from concept to manufacture for these specialized drugs.

Antidepressants

Chronic pain can lead to depression, and the use of prescribed antidepressants can help treat the symptoms of depression and also help relieve chronic pain and improve your sleep. They are more often used to treat the chronic pain and poor sleep of fibromyalgia than of arthritis. Dosage in this case is generally lower than that used to treat depression.

Antidepressants work by blocking the reuptake of one or more *neurotransmitters* responsible for relaying pain messages by the brain.

These medications include:

- Prozac (fluoxetine)

- Lexapro (escitalopram)

- Celexa (citalopram)

- Zoloft (sertraline)

- Paxil (paroxetine)

- Cymbalta (duloxetine Hcl)

- Wellbutrin (bupropion)

def•i•ni•tion

Neurotransmitters are chemicals released by the body's cells. Their function is to transmit neurological information from one cell to another.

Antidepressants that target two neurotransmitters (serotonin and norepinephrine) are called SNRIs—serotonin-norepinephrine reuptake inhibitors or simply, dual inhibitors. Cymbalta (duloxetine) and Effexor (venlafaxine) fall into this category.

An earlier class of antidepressants, the tricyclics, are still prescribed in some cases to aid in achieving restorative sleep in patients with chronic pain. Elavil (amitriptyline) and nortriptyline are tricyclic antidepressants used in low doses at bedtime to improve the quality of sleep.

Topical Pain Relievers

Topical pain relievers are rubs, sprays, creams, balms, lotions, gels, patches, ointments, and other products that are applied to the skin to provide temporary relief of minor muscle or joint pain. They are typically used when only a few joints are affected. Some topicals are used to treat skin conditions associated with certain types of arthritis.

Many topical creams and ointments are available over the counter. Those that contain combinations of salicylates essentially numb the nerve endings in the skin and interfere with their ability to sense pain. These include Aspercreme, Bengay, and Sportscreme, which contains trolamine salicylate, a chemical similar to aspirin.

Precautions

Capsaicin is the chemical found in hot chili peppers. When first used, it may cause a stinging or burning sensation, which usually subsides with continued applications.

Other topicals contain irritants, such as capsaicin (Zostrix), which stimulate nerve endings in the skin, causing sensations of cold, warmth, or itching that act as pain distracters.

It may take one to two weeks for a topical to achieve maximum effectiveness. Local anesthetics added to topicals work by numbing the area.

Muscle Relaxants

Muscle relaxants may be used to treat muscle spasms, pain, and stiffness. These medications generally act on the central nervous system. They can be prescribed for short-term use for muscle pain or for long-term application in patients with fibromyalgia who experience chronic muscle spasms. Several muscle relaxants are commonly prescribed:

- Robaxin (methocarbamol).

- Soma (carisoprodol).

- Flexeril (cyclobenzaprine). An additional benefit of Flexeril is improved quality of sleep, especially stage 4 sleep.

- Skelaxin (metaxalone). Skelaxin is the least likely of these medications to cause daytime drowsiness.

Other Drug Issues

Beyond the considerations of finding the right medication and discovering the best dosage to treat your symptoms, there are other matters of importance. Cost is, of course, a primary concern, especially when insurance plans do not cover the entire cost of the drug. There are other issues as well.

Alcohol and Medications

Whether you are taking prescription medications or over-the-counter medications, read the labels carefully and ask your physician or pharmacist if you should abstain from alcohol while taking them. Serious and potentially fatal complications can result from mixing certain drugs and alcohol.

Acetaminophen (Tylenol) and methotrexate are two drugs that do not interact well with alcohol, as the combination increases the risk of severe liver damage. NSAIDs mixed with alcohol can increase your risk of developing stomach ulcers.

Alcohol can interfere with both the quantity and quality of your sleep, resulting in increased fatigue and pain the next day. Alcohol may also interact with sleep medications, so it is important to tell your doctor how much alcohol you routinely consume. This is an area where honesty is essential. And there are other concerns regarding consumption of alcohol:

♦ Risk factor for gout

♦ Increased risk of osteoporosis

♦ Contributor to weight gain, which places added strain on inflamed joints

♦ Potential for elevating liver function tests, which may impact the dosage prescribed for your medications

Buying Prescription Medications Outside the United States

The Food and Drug Administration (FDA) is charged with ensuring the purity and safety of drugs in the United States. Its jurisdiction stops at the border, however, so you should be advised that purchasing your medications from foreign sources is not without risk.

While many people have purchased perfectly fine drugs at a cost savings in Canada, Mexico, or other foreign countries, similar packaging and appearance are not always indicators that the drug in question is the same as the one available in the United States. Production standards, including cleanliness and quality control, are highly

Consultation

Many older medications used for treating arthritis are now available as generics. These usually work as well as the branded products and result in significant cost savings.

variable. Additionally, you have no guarantees that the drug you are purchasing is in fact the drug you require, and you have no recourse should problems arise.

Buying Medications over the Internet

The Internet has become the premier marketplace for every commodity imaginable, and that includes drugs. However, quality control is not guaranteed, and you may not even receive the medication you ordered unless you purchase from a reputable site. An online pharmacist should be available to conduct appropriate oversight and answer any questions you may have.

Be aware that the U.S. Department of Justice Drug Enforcement Agency (DEA) has issued a consumer warning regarding the purchase of controlled substances over the Internet without a valid prescription from your physician. The criteria used to establish this validity is the existence of an actual doctor-patient relationship. In most instances, this requires a physical examination. Internet sites with "cyber-docs" who prescribe drugs based upon information submitted by online questionnaires do not fulfill the requirement for a real doctor-patient relationship.

To be sure the website you are planning to use is legitimate, consult the National Association of Boards of Pharmacy before you buy. Their website is www.nabp.net.

Sharing Medications

It may be tempting, especially when cost of drugs is a concern, to share your meds or to try someone else's. However, this can be dangerous—and even life-threatening. There is a potential for drug interactions, allergic reactions, or no reaction to the medication at all. Always consult your physician before taking any medication that has not been prescribed for you.

The Least You Need to Know

- Several classes of drugs are used to treat arthritis.

- NSAIDs are both anti-inflammatory agents and analgesics.

- Pure pain relievers such as Tylenol and narcotics do not help relieve inflammation.

- Doubling up on medications within a class of drugs can be dangerous.

- Buying your medications outside the United States or over the Internet can be risky.

Chapter 10

Surgical Interventions and Other Procedures

In This Chapter

- Expanding your treatment options
- Repairing cartilage damage
- Open versus arthroscopic surgeries
- Total joint replacements

At some point you may find that your medications just aren't providing the relief you need. Pain becomes a constant companion and loss of mobility a daily frustration. When you've tried all the recommended lifestyle changes and nothing seems to be helping, it may be time to consider surgery. In this chapter, you'll learn about the surgical procedures available for treating arthritis.

When to Consider Surgery

Several factors enter into the decision to have surgery, and you'll need to weigh each of them carefully. First, you'll discover that prescription and over-the-counter medications have maximum recommended doses. Once the upper dosage limits have been reached, serious and even potentially lethal health risks are possible. If you find that the medication dosages that initially gave you relief are no longer effective, continually upping your intake is not advisable. You may need to consider other options.

Second, though physical therapy can be of enormous benefit in keeping your joints functioning and increasing your range of motion, it has its limits. It can only do so much toward restoring mobility and improving range of motion for damaged joints. Physical therapy works with what you have. If cartilage damage has resulted in bone erosions in your joints, physical therapy cannot put healthy cartilage back or treat the erosions.

Consultation

Cartilage transplants have been mostly done on younger patients who have suffered knee injuries. It's not yet determined whether this kind of surgery benefits patients with osteoarthritis. These transplants are known by a variety of names, including autologous chondrocyte implantation, chondroplasty, and the Carticel approach.

Finally, losing excess weight and maintaining a program of mild to moderate exercise can bring you many benefits, but arthritis, particularly osteoarthritis, is a chronic, often progressive disease with no cure at this time. Healthy lifestyle changes can help you manage symptoms but work primarily to slow down the disease process.

Taking all these factors into consideration, you and your rheumatologist and orthopedic surgeon will decide when it's time to choose surgery. You'll weigh the benefits against the risks and educate yourself about the procedure or procedures that may benefit you. Ultimately, the final decision is yours. It will be up to you to make an informed decision as to what's best for you and your particular form of arthritis.

Removal of Joint Fluid

Removal of joint fluid, a procedure known as arthrocentesis, is both a diagnostic tool and a procedure to treat pain and inflammation. It's generally used to treat both osteoarthritis and rheumatoid arthritis.

As a diagnostic tool, arthrocentesis is used to determine the cause of joint swelling, which may be rheumatoid arthritis, gout, or infection. To treat inflammation with arthrocentesis, a doctor will remove excess joint fluid and then inject corticosteroids directly into the joint. Removal of the fluid and injecting cortisone usually decreases pain and improves joint mobility.

The knee, shoulder, ankle, and wrist joints particularly lend themselves to arthrocentesis. Your doctor may also call this procedure joint fluid aspiration, a joint tap, or synovial fluid aspiration.

How It's Done

Except for hip procedures, arthrocentesis can be done either in a doctor's office or a hospital. The physician first cleans the skin surface with an antiseptic solution. Then a local anesthetic is applied to the joint. This anesthetic can be delivered by injection, as a topical freezing liquid, or by both methods. A sterile needle and syringe are used to draw out the joint fluid. Drawing out the fluid is called aspiration.

Corticosteroids can then be injected into the joint to help provide pain relief and to reduce inflammation and swelling. After the procedure, the needle is withdrawn and a sterile dressing or strip is applied to the site. If there is any uncertainty about the proper diagnosis or the possibility of infection, the fluid may be sent to the lab for analysis.

The joint fluid can undergo a variety of tests to determine white blood cell count and the presence of crystals, protein, or glucose. It can also be *cultured* to detect the presence of infection. These tests may help determine the type of arthritis involved.

def•i•ni•tion

A **culture** is the process of growing microorganisms in a growth medium. It's done in a medical laboratory. Any body tissue or fluid can be evaluated in a laboratory by this method to detect and identify infectious agents.

Benefits, Risks, and Complications

If the joint is inflamed, removing the fluid also takes the white blood cells that are present in that fluid. Those white blood cells produce enzymes that, in excess, can harm the joint.

There may be some bruising at the site of the procedure and some minor bleeding into the joint, along with loss of pigment at the site of the needle entry. Infection of the joint, called septic arthritis, is a very rare but serious complication.

If corticosteroids have been injected into the joint, there may be short-term inflammation in the joint due to the crystallization of the medication, shrinkage or atrophy of the skin at the injection site, or loss of pigment. An increase in blood sugar levels for a day or two is an uncommon complication that may be of concern in patients with diabetes.

Removing the Joint Lining

In cases of inflammatory arthritis (such as rheumatoid arthritis, psoriatic arthritis, or juvenile arthritis), the joint lining, called the synovium, becomes inflamed and overgrows. This overgrowth is an abnormal immune response in which the body mistakes its own cartilage for a foreign substance and attacks it.

The synovium normally produces just the right amount of synovial fluid to lubricate the joint; an overgrown synovium, however, produces too much fluid. In too great a quantity, enzymes in this fluid can erode the cartilage at the surface of the joint where the bones meet. The loss of cartilage eventually causes joint damage, pain, and stiffness.

If your inflammatory arthritis has not responded to a six- to twelve-month course of treatment with medication, your rheumatologist may refer you to an orthopedic surgeon to have the inflamed joint lining removed, a procedure known as a synovectomy. This is usually done when only one or two joints are persistently inflamed. Inflammation in multiple joints is usually treated by systemic medications. Common sites for synovectomy include elbows, wrists, fingers, hips, knees, and ankles.

How It's Done

A synovectomy is a procedure to remove inflamed tissue (the word part -*ectomy* means "removal"). Depending on the location of the joint involved, your surgeon may opt for either an arthroscopic procedure (see the next section) or open surgery.

Researchers wondered if there were any significant differences in results between these two surgical methods. In studying the results of arthroscopic and open synovectomy of the elbow in patients with early rheumatoid arthritis, they found no significant differences between the overall clinical results of the methods. The study was published in the *Journal of Bone and Joint Surgery* (2006).

Another study considered the results of open synovectomy in patients with early rheumatoid arthritis involving the knuckles (called the metacarpophalangeal joints). These joints are important in all gripping motions. Researchers analyzed the outcomes of 252 patients. They found that after an average of almost seven years, patients reported relief with regard to joint mobility in 89 percent of cases, with regard to swelling in 87 percent of cases, and with regard to pain relief in 97 percent of cases. The conclusion was that open synovectomy results in very good long-term benefits. The study was reported in *Zeitschrift für Orthopädie und ihre Grenzgebiete* (2000).

Since both arthroscopic and open surgery can produce good outcomes, talk with your surgeon to see which approach will be best for your type of joint involvement.

Benefits, Risks, and Complications

There are several benefits to synovectomy. First, it may provide immediate pain relief and reduce swelling, although this can be temporary. It may also slow cartilage loss and erosions of the involved bones. Although the inflamed synovium is likely to grow back at some point, that may not be for five to ten years.

Another positive is the low complication rate with synovectomy. Risks include those associated with any surgery and the use of anesthesia. There may also be some bleeding within the joint along with a slight risk of infection. If symptoms return, including inflammation and decreased range of motion, additional surgery may be required.

If you have open surgery, your surgeon may refer you to physical therapy to address post-operative stiffness, which is more common after open surgery than arthroscopic surgery.

Consultation

Researchers are studying whether cartilage transplants, which have been performed mostly on patients who have suffered knee injuries, may be a treatment option for patients with osteoarthritis.

Arthroscopy

Arthroscopy may be a familiar term to you. It usually refers to an outpatient surgery that promotes pain relief by removing loose or damaged cartilage from the knee, a procedure known as debridement. Arthroscopy is used to treat osteoarthritis, inflammatory arthritis, and infectious arthritis.

When arthritis causes the joint lining (synovium) to become inflamed (a condition called synovitis), arthroscopy permits the surgeon to see that inflammation and to remove the inflamed lining. The term literally means "to look within the joint."

Arthroscopy was originally a diagnostic tool used to gather information prior to standard open surgery. Today, thanks to significant improvements and developments in the tools used for arthroscopy, the procedure can be used to also treat a variety of conditions.

Each year more than 650,000 arthroscopic knee procedures are performed in the United States, and about half of the patients who undergo the surgery report pain relief. Shoulders and knees are the usual sites for arthroscopic surgery, because they are large enough for the instruments required. It is possible to perform arthroscopic surgery on hips, elbows, ankles, and wrists, but the smaller joint spaces there may make this option more difficult.

How It's Done

You'll either report to an outpatient surgery or be checked into the hospital as a patient. You'll receive an anesthetic—either general, which means you'll be asleep for the entire procedure, or local, which will just numb the surgical area.

An incision about 1 centimeter (0.4 inch) in length is made and a tiny video camera is inserted through the incision, allowing your surgeon a clear view of the inside of the joint. The camera is attached to a fiber-optic light source and the image is projected onto a television monitor in the operating room. The surgeon injects water into the joint to expand it and to allow more maneuvering room while he removes the damaged tissue.

The incision will be covered with a sterile dressing. If you've had a general anesthetic, you'll be transferred to a recovery area until the anesthesia has worn off and you are fully conscious. The incision will take several days to heal and the joint will take several weeks to achieve maximum healing.

You will not be able to drive yourself home and will need to have someone transport you. You'll be given discharge instructions on how to care for the incision and what to look for if there are problems and a date for a follow-up appointment with your surgeon. You'll also most likely be given a copy of the video of your surgery to watch at home. It's a fascinating process.

At your follow-up appointment, any sutures will be removed and you may be referred to physical therapy to help you gain strength and function in your joint.

Benefits, Risks, and Complications

Arthroscopic surgery is considered less invasive than open surgery. It's generally less painful and often is more cost-effective. Since it's often done on an outpatient basis, you're usually able to go home the same day instead of spending the night at the hospital, as you're likely to do with open surgery. You will most likely be able to resume most of your normal activities within a few days of surgery.

As with any surgical procedure, there are risks which include infection, blood clots, or an adverse reaction to the anesthetic. There may be some swelling at the incision site and some bleeding may occur. Instrument breakage during the surgery is a very uncommon possibility; complications occur in less than 1 percent of all arthroscopic procedures.

While arthroscopic surgery to repair torn cartilage or a ligament is of clear benefit in younger individuals with acute athletic and other injuries, its use as an effective treatment for knee osteoarthritis pain has been questioned.

In 2002, researchers began a two-year study at a Veterans Affairs hospital in Houston, Texas. For the study, researchers divided 180 participants into 3 groups. The first group had the arthroscopic procedure, the second group received a saline cleansing of the interior knee, and the third received no treatment, except for a small incision to make it appear they had undergone arthroscopic knee surgery. The third group was called the "sham surgery" group.

The researchers found no difference in outcomes among the three groups and concluded that arthroscopic knee surgery was no more effective than the sham surgery. They suggested that the placebo effect was the reason the participants experienced pain relief. The study appeared in the *New England Journal of Medicine*.

In cases of advanced arthritis, knee arthroscopy will likely not provide much benefit. However, as a means of trimming damaged cartilage, it may provide pain relief by reducing inflammation or preventing locking. The average recovery period for arthroscopy is four to six weeks. This compares to a three- to nine-month recovery period for a total knee replacement, so it may be worth considering surgery early on.

Consultation

The placebo effect occurs when patients experience relief from symptoms, and sometimes a cure, in the absence of any real treatment. The mind believes that treatment has occurred and the body accepts that belief and acts upon it. It is a real phenomenon and only partly understood.

Joint Replacement

In joint replacement surgery, a severely damaged joint is replaced with an artificial one to restore function and provide pain relief. It is generally considered when medications and lifestyle changes have not helped. Joint replacement surgery is primarily used to treat osteoarthritis. It may also be performed to treat inflammatory arthritis.

Joint replacement surgery is called arthroplasty or total joint arthroplasty. It's primarily performed on the knees and hips, although the shoulder, elbow, ankle, and fingers are also candidates. The American Academy of Orthopaedic Surgeons (www.2aaos. org) reports that by 2030, orthopedic surgeons in the United States could be performing more than 571,100 primary total hip arthroplasties and an estimated 3.48 million total knee arthroplasties.

There are two types of joint replacement surgery: joint resection and interpositional reconstruction.

In joint resection, the surgeon removes a portion of bone from the affected joint. This enlarges the space between the bone and the socket and results in improved range of motion along with pain relief. Scar tissue eventually forms around the area, creating a false joint. Joint resection is used frequently to treat rheumatoid arthritis in the foot.

def•i•ni•tion

Fascia is a thin layer of connective tissue that covers or connects the muscles or inner organs of the body.

For interpositional reconstruction, both bones that make up the joint are reshaped and a prosthetic disk is inserted between them to function the way healthy cartilage would—to keep the bones from rubbing together. The prosthesis may be plastic, metal, ceramic, or formed from body tissue, such as skin, muscle, or *fascia*. If interpositional reconstruction fails, total joint replacement may be necessary.

Standard thinking has been that arthroplasty should only be performed on severely affected joints that have been deteriorating for quite some time. Especially in younger patients, the approach has been to wait, since the joints will eventually need to be replaced and these subsequent surgeries may have more potential for complications. But now some medical experts are encouraging patients to have the procedure done earlier, as recovery may be more complete if the patient has not become severely disabled.

How It's Done

Joint replacement is performed under either general or local (numbing a specific area) anesthesia by an orthopedic surgeon at a hospital. Orthopedic hospitals and medical centers that perform larger numbers of arthroplastic procedures tend to have higher success rates than do general hospitals.

For joint resection, the surgeon removes the damaged joint surfaces and replaces them with plastic and metal prostheses. The more bone and more ligaments that remain, the more stable the joint will be. Your surgeon will try to preserve as much ligament attachment as possible.

There are two methods available for attaching the prosthesis to the adjoining bone: cemented and cementless. A cemented method is generally used in older patients who have thinner bones. In a cementless implant, either the prosthesis is coated with a porous material that allows bone to grow into and adhere to the prosthesis or the joint components are specially fitted to press into the bone for a tight fit (called a press-fit). This process is generally used in patients under age 65 who will probably need revision arthroplasty in the future (see the next section). If the bone doesn't grow into the porous material, however, additional surgery to cement the prosthesis may be necessary.

Consultation

The knee joint is the largest joint in the body. It's formed where the lower part of the thighbone (femur) joins the upper part of the shinbone (tibia) and the kneecap (patella).

After surgery, you are likely to remain in the hospital an average of three days. You'll begin a physical therapy program right away to help aid in your recovery. It will take about six weeks to rebuild adjoining muscle and strengthen the surrounding ligaments.

If you are having both knees replaced, you will usually not have them done together. You will wait until your first knee has healed before undergoing the second procedure. The exception might be a younger person in good health who is capable of tolerating the longer bilateral surgery and can't afford to take as much time off from work as would be required for two separate procedures.

Benefits, Risks, and Complications

Benefits of joint replacement surgery include relief from pain and improved range of motion; however, an artificial joint, for all its ability to help functioning, is not equivalent to the original and may not have the complete range of motion of a healthy, normal joint. As well, artificial joints can eventually wear out and they can loosen. The average life span for an artificial joint is between 10 and 20 years.

The risks of joint replacement surgery include those associated with any surgery, including reaction to anesthesia, post-operative infection, and blood clots. Other complications and side effects include thigh pain, hip dislocation (a 3.1 percent chance after a first procedure, increasing to 14.4 percent after a second procedure), uneven leg lengths, nerve damage, urinary tract infections, delayed healing, and allergic reactions to the metal used.

More serious risks include a 1 percent chance of death within three months of an initial procedure and a 2.6 percent chance after a second procedure. The risk is highest in the first three months after surgery.

Precautions

The FDA considers artificial joints to be medical devices. They can't be rushed to the marketplace until the FDA has given its approval.

Long-term complications include failure of the implant due to bone damage caused by the release of tiny particles from the prosthesis. There is a rare possibility of an autoimmune response if loose particles released by the implant trigger the immune system.

Generally those at highest risk for complications are the elderly, men, African Americans, and those with other serious medical conditions.

Revision Total Joint Replacement

Revision total joint replacement, also known as revision arthroplasty, is a second surgery that's required to replace a joint replacement that has worn out or failed. There may be more than one cause for joint failure. These factors can be interrelated and include infection, bone loss (osteolysis), or joint loosening. When a replacement joint becomes loose, it may be because it wasn't placed correctly during surgery or because the patient made too many demands on the new joint.

Osteolysis can occur when the prosthesis is loose, is infected, or was incorrectly positioned during surgery. It can also be a result of the accumulation of wear particles from a plastic prosthesis. Newer plastics may solve the latter problem.

Your orthopedic surgeon will need to evaluate your individual situation before making a recommendation. If there is a problem with just one part, then not all of them may need to be replaced. There are essentially three options for revision joint replacement: a total joint replacement, a new prosthesis, or a prosthesis specifically designed for your particular situation.

Revision joint replacement is more complicated than the original procedure, and the results are not as consistent. The type of surgery generally depends upon whether the problem is within the socket cavity or space (a contained defect) or outside the socket cavity (an uncontained defect).

If the defect is contained, small bone grafts, cement, or oversized cementless implants can be used to repair it. If the defect is uncontained, a large bone graft or implants may be necessary to restore bone.

If small amounts of bone are needed, these may be taken from bone removed during the surgery or from another location in your body, such as the pelvis. If larger amounts are needed, donor bone (obtained from cadavers) may be required.

A second arthroplastic procedure does come with increased risks for complications. The surgical field is bigger, more bone must be cut, more blood may be lost, and you will be under anesthesia for a longer period of time. Additionally, the potential for complications increases overall with age.

> **Straight Talk**
>
> When my hip replacement loosened, the pain became almost unbearable. I was forced to use a wheelchair or a walker. I decided to have the revision surgery and can now look forward to getting around on my own and getting back to living.
>
> —Markey, age 61, osteoarthritis patient

Realigning the Bones

Surgery to realign the bones is called osteotomy. It's used to treat osteoarthritis of the knee and hip and may be a good alternative to total joint replacement.

This surgery can provide pain relief and also slow the progression of osteoarthritis by redirecting stress away from the damaged portion of the bone and toward healthier tissue. It can be performed in younger people with osteoarthritis when joint replacement surgery isn't indicated. It's also used in heavier adults under age 60.

If you have uneven damage to a joint, if just one side of a joint is affected, or if you have a correctable deformity and lack of inflammation, you may be a candidate for this surgery.

How It's Done

Osteotomy is done under general anesthesia by an orthopedic surgeon in the hospital. In a knee osteotomy, the bone is cut and a portion may be removed to permit the weight to shift to the healthy side of the joint. This stabilizes the knee and reduces the pain that results from bearing weight on damaged cartilage. Improving knee alignment may require the surgeon to reshape the shinbone (tibia) or the thighbone (femur). The surgeon may need to move healthy cartilage and bone to accomplish a successful repositioning.

The most commonly performed knee osteotomy is done on a knee that angles inward (knock-kneed). In this case, the surgeon treats arthritis of the inside compartment of the knee. If the knee angles outward (bow-legged), the surgeon treats arthritis of the outside compartment of the knee.

After surgery, the joint may be held in place with a cast, staples, or internal plates. The knee may not appear symmetrical after surgery, and eventually a total knee replacement may be required. A cast or splint is worn for four to eight weeks.

In a hip osteotomy, the surgeon cuts the bones of the hip joint, repositions them, and fixes them in their new position. Healthy cartilage is placed in the joint's weight-bearing area. Finally, the joint is reconstructed to achieve a more normal position.

Benefits, Risks, and Complications

Outcomes for osteotomy are generally good, with full recovery taking from six to twelve months. A successful osteotomy can delay a total joint replacement up to 10 years.

There may be pain after surgery and extensive physical therapy is generally required. Potential risks associated with this surgery include bones that fail to heal correctly, blood clots, bleeding into the joint, infection, inflammation, and nerve damage.

Fusing the Joints

Joint fusion is an alternative to joint replacement surgery and is performed when joint replacement isn't an option. It works by fusing the two bones on each side of the joint and thus eliminating the joint—the source of the pain!

Joint fusion, also called arthrodesis, is most commonly done on the spine, so it can bear weight without pain. It's also done with the small bones of the hands and feet. The drawback to this surgery is that the joint is no longer flexible. A fused finger or ankle will not bend. Joint fusion is used to treat osteoarthritis, spondylarthropathy, or inflammatory arthritis.

Results of arthrodesis include pain relief, restored skeletal stability, and improved spinal alignment in individuals with advanced arthritis.

In a joint fusion surgery, the surgeon performs a bone graft under general or local anesthetic. She takes bone from another part of the body or from a bone bank at the hospital and inserts it between the two bones being fused to stimulate the fusion.

Then metal plates, screws, or wires may be used to close the joint and position the bones next to each other. Over time, the bones heal and fuse to become one.

Spinal Fusion and Instrumentation

In spinal fusion, a bone graft is used to create a bridge that allows two opposing bony surfaces to meet and grow together. Spinal instrumentation is a surgical procedure to straighten and stabilize the spine after spinal fusion.

In spinal instrumentation, hooks, rods, and wires are surgically attached to the spine to redistribute stress on the spine and keep it in correct alignment. Spinal instrumentation surgically implants titanium, titanium alloy, stainless steel, or nonmetallic devices directly into the spine. It's a permanent solution to spinal instability.

The first spinal fusion was performed almost 90 years ago. Spinal instrumentation was developed by Dr. Paul Harrington in the late 1950s to help keep children stricken with polio from developing spinal deformities.

How It's Done

Spinal fusion and instrumentation is performed while you're under general anesthesia. The orthopedic surgeon first strips the muscles away from the area to be fused. Next, the surface of the bone is peeled away. The stripping of the bone helps stimulate the graft to fuse. Then a piece of bone is taken from your pelvis and placed alongside the area to be fused. The rods, hooks, and wires are inserted and the incision is closed.

Healing may take from six to eight months and in certain instances you may be required to wear a body cast. After the cast is removed, you may need to wear a back brace for some time. During your recovery period, you'll definitely have decreased mobility.

Benefits, Risks, and Complications

After arthrodesis, a fused joint is more able to bear weight, more stable, and less painful. Flexibility, however, is no longer possible.

Risks include pain at the site of bone fusion, failure of the fusion, breakage of metal implants, nerve injury, and infection. Serious risks of spinal fusion include nerve damage and the possibility of paralysis. Long-term complications include instrumentation breakage, which requires additional surgery.

If you have had spinal instrumentation, you will need to avoid contact sports and situations that put excess strain on your spine for the rest of your life.

The Least You Need to Know

- Surgery should be considered only after all other treatment protocols have been exhausted.

- Arthroscopic surgery is less invasive than open surgery and may provide good results for some types of arthritis.

- The average lifespan of an artificial joint is 10 to 20 years.

- Surgery can relieve pain and inflammation but cannot cure arthritis, which is a chronic and progressive disease.

- Surgical procedures can involve removing, reshaping, repositioning, and replacing bone.

11

Complementary Therapies: Products

In This Chapter

- ◆ Adding supplements to your arthritis treatment protocol
- ◆ Seeking out purity and quality
- ◆ Natural doesn't always mean safe
- ◆ Super foods that can cure

Long before medical laboratories began churning out pills and capsules, herbs and foods were used to treat disease. Especially in Eastern cultures, this form of traditional medicine has a long and respected history. It's only been fairly recently, however, that the Western medical tradition has embraced some of these remedies.

Originally these treatments were considered alternatives to standard medical treatment, but as their uses and benefits have become known, many of these supplements, foods, and herbs have been incorporated into mainstream medicine. A new field of medicine, referred to as complementary or integrative medicine, now incorporates these time-honored approaches to healing into modern Western practices.

Dietary Supplements

Grocery stores, pharmacies, and health food stores stock a variety of dietary supplements. You can learn about them through infomercials on television, magazine advertisements, and word-of-mouth testimonials from friends and relatives. Some people swear by them, and others find no benefit. Some research studies find that they work, and other studies find that they don't.

What are dietary supplements? According to the Dietary Supplement Health and Education Act of 1994, a dietary supplement is a product other than tobacco that ...

♦ Is labeled as a dietary supplement.

♦ Is taken as a pill, liquid, capsule, or tablet.

♦ Contains one or more dietary ingredients, such as vitamins, minerals, herbs or other botanicals, amino acids, or substances such as enzymes, organ tissues, *glandulars*, and *metabolites*.

def•i•ni•tion

Glandulars are extracts of animal organs that contain hormones and other substances found in those organs. Not all of these substances have been medically identified. **Metabolites** are any of the substances produced by the metabolism—the entire range of biochemical processes occurring within the body.

This definition takes in a vast amount of territory, and while supplements have been defined, they aren't regulated by the Food and Drug Administration (FDA). The FDA considers herbs and supplements neither food nor drugs, so it does not have standards regarding their production. Only when a product has proven to be unsafe does this government agency become involved. This limited oversight can have serious consequences for the unwary consumer.

Several dietary supplements are used to treat the pain and inflammation of arthritis.

Glucosamine and Chondroitin

Glucosamine and chondroitin have only been tested for and recommended for treatment of osteoarthritis. Their use is *not* indicated to treat rheumatoid or other types of arthritis. What's the truth behind these supplements? Are they safe? Do they work?

What They Are

Glucosamine (glucosamine hydrochloride) and chondroitin (chondroitin sulfate) are natural substances believed to be both the building blocks of cartilage and stimulants that cause the body to make new cartilage. They have been widely used as supplements in Europe over the past decade. This has spurred research in the United States on their efficacy in treating osteoarthritis.

Some studies have shown that glucosamine may improve joint flexibility and relieve osteoarthritis pain. Glucosamine has mild anti-inflammatory properties and stimulates cartilage to produce collagen and proteoglycans, substances that keep your joints healthy.

Chondroitin is a carbohydrate. It's believed that chondroitin inhibits the enzymes responsible for the breakdown of cartilage. Chondroitin and glucosamine are frequently included together in supplement form.

How They Work

Osteoarthritis causes the cartilage in joints to break down, and glucosamine and chondroitin may help the body repair that damaged cartilage. Researchers do not know yet exactly how these supplements work.

Effectiveness

Glucosamine has been extensively studied for its benefits and different studies have had different results. A study published in the March 15, 2000, issue of the *Journal of the American Medical Association* (JAMA) found that glucosamine had a moderate effect on pain relief and also improved mobility.

Additionally, the study found that chondroitin had a significantly positive effect. Researchers concluded that these supplements may slow the progression of cartilage loss in osteoarthritis. They found these supplements to be at least as effective as ibuprofen (Advil, Motrin). Several other studies also found these supplements to be beneficial:

- In a three-year study involving 212 people with osteoarthritis in their knees, researchers found that patients who took glucosamine experienced far less joint deterioration than those who did not. Patients who were given glucosamine also reported decreased joint pain. The study was reported in *The Lancet* (January 24, 2001).

- A study published in the *Archives of Internal Medicine* (July 14, 2003) showed that glucosamine and chondroitin significantly improved

Precautions

Glucosamine and chondroitin need to be taken for at least one month to have the best therapeutic results.

symptoms of osteoarthritis and also improved joint mobility for one in five patients studied.

♦ Research presented at the 2006 American College of Rheumatology annual meeting suggested that chondroitin may prevent joint narrowing in patients with knee osteoarthritis.

On the other side of the coin, however, in 2006, the *New England Journal of Medicine* published the results of a major six-month trial sponsored by the National Institutes of Health (NIH). The trial compared the effects of glucosamine and chondroitin (alone and in combination) with the COX-2 inhibitor celecoxib (Celebrex) in nearly 1,600 patients with knee osteoarthritis. They also compared these supplements with the effects of a placebo (an inactive substance).

The results indicated that for most patients, neither glucosamine nor chondroitin alone were more effective than the placebo in relieving the pain of knee osteoarthritis. For patients with moderate-to-severe pain, however, a combination of glucosamine and chondroitin was significantly more effective. They found that Celebrex worked best for patients with mild pain.

So what does this mean? It means that research will continue trying to discover whether glucosamine and chondroitin, either alone or together, can actually halt the progression of knee OA. Also to be determined is the long-term safety of using these supplements.

Safety Considerations

As with other dietary supplements, the purity of glucosamine and chondroitin products sold in pharmacies, health food stores, and supermarkets is not regulated by the Food and Drug Administration. Always check with your physician before deciding to take any supplement, as they may have adverse reactions with other medications or supplements you are taking. If you decide to add glucosamine and chondroitin to your arthritis treatment plan, there are a few other things to be aware of:

♦ Glucosamine is manufactured from the shells of shellfish and chondroitin is made from shark cartilage. If you have allergies to shellfish, consult your physician before using these supplements.

♦ These supplements may raise blood sugar levels, which may be a concern if you have diabetes.

 ♦ These supplements have a blood-thinning effect, which may be a concern if you are taking blood-thinning medications (anticoagulants).

 ♦ These supplements are not recommended for children or women who are pregnant or who could become pregnant.

The most commonly reported side effects include nausea, diarrhea or constipation, heartburn, and increased intestinal gas.

Truth in Labeling

This is truly a case of caveat emptor—buyer beware. Because supplements aren't regulated by the FDA, you really don't know what you're getting inside that bottle. Studies have found that the amount of active ingredients may not be what is claimed on the label. In some cases, you're not getting any of what you're paying for!

A report carried on www.msnbc.msn.com on April 11, 2007, revealed some startling information from ConsumerLab.com, an independent company that evaluates health and nutrition products and publishes reviews of their findings. ConsumerLab.com had chosen 20 joint supplements and had them tested by independent laboratories. Of the supplements tested, 40 percent were found not to contain what the labels indicated. Of 11 brands claiming to contain chondroitin, 8 failed to meet standards. Several established brands were among the failures:

 ♦ Karuna Chondroitin Sulfate contained only half the chondroitin stated on the label.

 ♦ Nature's Plus Ultra Maximum Strength Chondroitin 600 contained no detectable chondroitin.

 ♦ Swanson Health Products Premium Brand Glucosamine & Chondroitin had only 8 percent of the promised chondroitin.

 ♦ Weil Glucosamine & Chondroitin contained the ingredients claimed, but they didn't break down quickly enough. The supplement would pass through a person's body without being absorbed.

There's more involved here than truth in labeling issues. Not only are you paying for a product that you aren't getting, but you're not getting the therapeutic benefit of the supplements.

Yet another concern in this unregulated market is that impurities or potential allergens may be present in the fillers and binders of pills. These may not be listed in the ingredients.

Consultation _____

Your rheumatologist and pharmacist are your best sources of information regarding the safety of supplements. To increase your chances of receiving what you're paying for, check with them for the names of reliable brands.

MSM

MSM, or methylsulfonylmethane, is another supplement used to treat arthritis. MSM occurs naturally in meats, fish, certain fruits, vegetables, and grains, but is destroyed with cooking. This odorless and tasteless natural sulfur compound is claimed to promote healthy connective tissue and joint function and may have pain-relieving and anti-inflammatory properties, as well. This may make MSM of some use for treating rheumatoid arthritis, osteoarthritis, gout, and fibromyalgia.

MSM hasn't been researched as thoroughly as glucosamine and chondroitin, although two small studies have suggested that MSM may reduce the joint pain of osteoarthritis. It hasn't been shown to preserve cartilage or to stop the progression of the disease or the destruction of the joints.

The Mayo Clinic reports that MSM is generally considered to be safe, although side effects may include diarrhea, skin rash, headache, mild cramps, stomach upset, and fatigue.

SAM-e

SAM-e (pronounced *Sammy*) is a synthetic form of a byproduct of an amino acid that occurs naturally in the human body. It helps produce hormones and cell membranes.

In Europe, this supplement has been available for several years as a prescription medicine to treat arthritis symptoms. It became available as an over-the-counter medication in the United States in 1999. SAM-e can be expensive and may not be covered by your insurance.

Some studies indicate that SAM-e may relieve the pain of osteoarthritis as well as non-steroidal anti-inflammatory drugs (NSAIDs) do. The Mayo Clinic reports that it also seems to have fewer side effects. At this time, there are no long-term studies showing the effects of taking SAM-e for extended periods.

Systemic Oral Enzymes

Enzymes have been used since biblical times to treat various illnesses, and they may help treat the symptoms of arthritis. Enzymes may prove to be safer alternatives to nonsteroidal anti-inflammatory drugs (NSAIDs). Enzymes such as bromelain, trypsin, papain, and rutin have been used in Europe for quite some time. They may be sold separately or in combinations (Wobenzym, Phlogenzym).

Studies seem to indicate that systemic oral enzymes may help the immune system become more efficient at clearing cellular debris, thus reducing inflammation. It appears that they can be taken indefinitely without negative consequences.

def•i•ni•tion

An **enzyme** is a protein that acts as a catalyst to speed up the body's biochemical reactions. Most of the body's functions require an enzyme to get started.

A six-month study of systemic oral enzymes was conducted at the Arizona Research and Education Center in 2001 with 240 patients with knee osteoarthritis. Systemic oral enzymes were found to be effective in relieving pain, reducing swelling, and aiding in joint mobility. No significant side effects were observed; however, symptoms returned when the enzymes were discontinued.

Botanicals

Products made from botanicals (plants or plant parts) can be marketed as herbal products, botanical products, or phytomedicines. Many botanicals meet the criteria for food supplements as outlined in the Dietary Supplement Health and Education Act of 1994.

Many of these products are marketed as "natural" and bear some investigating as to what this actually means.

Herbs can truly be Mother Nature's medicine chest. The early Native Americans discovered that the bark of the willow tree, when chewed, was an effective pain reliever.

Precautions _____

Just because a product is natural doesn't ensure that it will be helpful in treating your arthritis or that it won't cause you any harm. Many natural products can be harmful, and some are lethal.

Today we know that the anti-inflammatory agent salicin, the word from which *aspirin* is derived, was the reason.

Many botanicals have been used across the centuries to treat the pain and inflammation of arthritis. Some are commonplace, and others may be unfamiliar to you. Herbs may interact with other herbs, supplements, or medications, however, so always check with your physician before embarking on a program of herbal remedies.

Ginger

The University of Maryland Medical Center is an excellent resource for information on botanicals used to treat arthritis. Ginger is one of these botanicals and has been used in many cultures over the centuries to treat arthritis.

It's an interesting-looking root—knobby and thick and light beige in color. Fresh ginger root is found in the produce section of your grocery store and dried ginger root may be packaged in tea bags, capsules, or tablets. It is also sold in a liquid form. Fresh ginger root is an anti-inflammatory and a COX-2 inhibitor.

A 2001 study of patients with knee osteoarthritis ("Effects of a ginger extract on knee pain in patients") found that an extract of ginger reduced pain both while standing and after walking. After six weeks of taking ginger, patients were able to cut back on their pain medications. The study was reported in *Arthritis and Rheumatism* (volume 44, issue 11, published online November 7, 2001).

Consultation _____

Co-author Neal's own practice was a study site for a ginger clinical trial. The "ginger burps" were very significant and patients could readily tell if they were in the treatment group or taking the placebo. No improvement was seen among the patients given ginger.

Side effects may include mild digestive upset. Ginger may also increase your risk of bleeding if you are taking blood thinners (anticoagulants), including aspirin. If you have gallstones, check with your physician before taking ginger supplements. Ginger may also alter the effects of some prescription and over-the-counter medications, so it's best to check with your pharmacist or physician.

As with dietary supplements, studies of botanicals may show opposite findings. One study found that ginger was no more effective than ibuprofen or a placebo in reducing symptoms of OA.

If you decide to give ginger a try to relieve your arthritis pain, the University of Maryland Medical Center advises taking 2 to 4 grams of fresh ginger juice, extract, or tea daily. Try rubbing topical ginger oil into painful joints, or apply fresh ginger root to painful joints in a warm poultice or compress.

Thunder God Vine

The National Institutes of Health reports that thunder god vine (*Tripterygium wilfordii*), also known as *lei gong teng*, has been used in China for its medicinal properties for more than 400 years.

This is not a plant that you want to gather on your own, even if your travels do take you to the Orient. It can cause severe side effects and can be poisonous if it's not carefully extracted from the skinned root. Other parts of the plant—including the leaves, flowers, and skin of the root—are highly poisonous and can cause death.

Side effects include diarrhea, upset stomach, hair loss, headache, menstrual changes, and skin rash. Thunder god vine has been found to decrease bone mineral density in women who take the herb for five or more years. If you are at risk for osteoporosis, check with your physician before considering thunder god vine.

In traditional Chinese medicine, thunder god vine is used to treat a variety of autoimmune and inflammatory conditions, including rheumatoid arthritis, systemic lupus erythematosus (SLE), ankylosing spondylitis, and psoriasis.

Results from a small study funded by the National Institute of Arthritis and Musculoskeletal and Skin Diseases (NIAMS) indicate that an oral extract of the herb may improve rheumatoid arthritis symptoms in some patients. A small study on thunder god vine applied to the skin also found benefits for rheumatoid arthritis symptoms.

Extracts prepared from the skinned root of the thunder god vine may be used in ointment form for rheumatoid arthritis or taken orally as a treatment for RA and lupus.

Turmeric

Turmeric (*Curcuma longa*) is an ancient ayurvedic herb with both culinary and medicinal uses (see Chapter 12). It has anti-inflammatory properties, and several modern studies tend to support its ability to alleviate the symptoms of arthritis, specifically improving morning stiffness and physical endurance.

Precautions

ConsumerLab.com found that lead contamination was a concern in turmeric supplements sold in capsule form. Additionally, in some cases the supplements tested lacked the stated ingredient amounts. These test results were reported in May 2008.

Curcumin, derived from turmeric, has both antioxidant and anti-inflammatory properties. A 2006 study found that curcumin may be of benefit for gout and pseudogout—the crystalline types of arthritis.

The November 2006 issue of *Arthritis & Rheumatism* published the results of a study of the effectiveness of turmeric as a treatment to reduce inflammation. Researchers recommended that clinical trials in humans be initiated to see if turmeric might be useful to treat arthritis symptoms. It is believed that turmeric is a natural COX-2 inhibitor.

Cat's Claw

The University of Maryland Medical Center describes cat's claw (*Uncaria tomentosa*), a woody vine native to the Amazon rainforest and other tropical areas of South and Central America, as a possible arthritis remedy. Hooklike thorns growing along the vine gave rise to the name. Both the bark and root of cat's claw have been used for centuries by South Americans, including the Inca, to treat osteoarthritis. The bark of the cat's claw vine is crushed to make a tea. It's also available in liquid and capsule form.

Research regarding the safety and effectiveness of cat's claw is limited, although one study found that it may help relieve the pain of knee OA without side effects.

Devil's Claw

This African plant (*Harpagophytum procumbens*) got its name from its fruit that resembles a clawlike hand. It has been used in Europe for nearly 300 years and for even longer in Africa.

How devil's claw might work to relieve the symptoms of arthritis is not yet known, although one study showed it was most effective in combination with nonsteroidal anti-inflammatory drugs (NSAIDs). Because of this, taking devil's claw may enable you to reduce the dose of NSAIDs you are taking.

Side effects include ringing in the ears, diarrhea, and decreases in appetite and taste. Since devil's claw may change your levels of stomach acids, you should not take this supplement if you have stomach ulcers. It may also be of concern if you are diabetic, as this herb may lower blood sugar levels.

Feverfew

Feverfew (*Tanacetum parthenium*), although a member of the sunflower family, is a much shorter relative. It is native to southeastern Europe and has been used for centuries in Europe as a remedy for headaches, arthritis, and fevers. The name *feverfew* means "fever reducer." It works as an anti-inflammatory agent.

The active agent in feverfew is parthenolide, which inhibits compounds that cause inflammation. Dried feverfew leaves are usually used as supplements, but all above-ground parts of the plant have medical value. The University of Maryland Medical Center advises that feverfew supplements are available fresh, freeze-dried, or dried and can be purchased in capsule, tablet, or liquid extract forms.

But though feverfew has documented anti-inflammatory properties, a human study conducted in 1989 concluded that feverfew was no more effective than a placebo in improving symptoms of rheumatoid arthritis. Further studies will help determine the effectiveness of feverfew.

The University of Maryland Medical Center advises that the side effects of feverfew range from mild to moderate:

- Gastrointestinal problems such as abdominal pain, indigestion, flatulence, and diarrhea
- Nausea
- Vomiting
- Nervousness
- Mouth ulcers, loss of taste, and swelling of the lips, tongue, and mouth

If you have allergies to chamomile, ragweed, or yarrow, you will likely be allergic to feverfew and should not take this supplement.

If you have a bleeding disorder or are taking blood-thinning medications, such as aspirin or warfarin, you should not take feverfew. It is not recommended for women who are pregnant or who may become pregnant or for children.

Feverfew should be discontinued gradually if you have been taking it for more than one week. Withdrawal symptoms include headache, anxiety, fatigue, muscle stiffness, and joint pain.

Autumn Crocus

This highly toxic plant (*Colchicum autumnale*) was used by the ancient Egyptians to treat gout. *Rodale's Illustrated Encyclopedia of Herbs* (Rodale Press, 1998) notes that today the alkaloid colchicine is extracted from the corm and the seeds of the plant and prescribed either in tablet form or intravenously to treat gout.

An overdose of the drug may cause nausea, vomiting, abdominal pains, extreme thirst, weak pulse, and coldness and pain in the extremities. The kidneys and blood vessels may be damaged.

Precautions _____

> Autumn crocus is one plant to leave alone to enjoy its beauty in the garden. All parts of the autumn crocus are poisonous, and though colchicine has therapeutic value, it is lethal even in small doses.

Yucca

The Mayo Clinic notes that yucca plants (*Agavaceae*) grow in the arid regions of North America. According to medicinal folklore, yucca contains compounds that help suppress certain intestinal microorganisms that may play a role in joint inflammation. This has yet to be proven: although scientific studies have validated many alternative and complementary therapies for arthritis, yucca, according to the Mayo Clinic, is not one of them.

Super Foods to the Rescue

Super foods are foods packed with antioxidants, vitamins, and minerals. They nourish the body and help the immune system stay strong and healthy. In the fight against arthritis, these foods can be powerful allies.

Salmon

Fish oils are the good oils. They are high in omega-3 fatty acids and help reduce inflammation. Salmon is an excellent source of omega-3 fatty acids and among the richest sources of healthy fats. (Cod liver oil is also included in this group.) If you suffer from rheumatoid arthritis, this is of interest to you.

It's really hard to go wrong with salmon. If you don't like salmon, shrimp also contains omega-3 fatty acids and vitamin C, along with other nutrients essential for general health, including iron and vitamin B_{12}.

Cheese

Arthritis is all about your joints, your joints are all about your bones, and cheese is all about providing calcium for those bones. Whether you prefer hard cheeses such as cheddar or softer cheeses such as Havarti, they are an excellent source of calcium to help promote bone health. In addition, cheese supplies protein to strengthen the muscles and other tissues that support your joints.

Green Peppers

A study presented in the *Annals of the Rheumatic Diseases* reported that people who consumed the lowest amounts of vitamin C–enriched foods were more than three times more likely to develop arthritis than those who consumed the highest amounts of vitamin C–enriched foods.

One green pepper contains 176 percent of your daily requirement for vitamin C. Green peppers are richer in vitamin C than oranges and grapefruit and are also good sources of vitamin B_6.

Straight Talk

Hippocrates, the famous Greek physician who gave us the Hippocratic Oath, also said, "Let food be your medicine."

Bananas

Bananas are also good sources of vitamin B_6, folate, and vitamin C. They're easily digestible and a great source of soluble fiber.

Extra-Virgin Olive Oil

You probably already cook with olive oil, but you may not be aware of its possible arthritis-fighting properties. Olive oil is a monounsaturated fat with antioxidant properties that may protect the body against inflammation. Monounsaturated fats lower your total cholesterol. They raise your good cholesterol (HDL) while decreasing levels of bad cholesterol (LDL).

In animal studies, rats with arthritis were fed diets high in various kinds of oils. The researchers found that both fish oil and olive oil prevented or helped reduce arthritis-related inflammation.

Green Tea

While green tea's effects on the symptoms of rheumatoid arthritis have not been researched in people, they have been studied in mice.

A study funded by the Arthritis Foundation and reported in the Proceedings of the National Academy of Sciences, found that the antioxidants found in green tea, known as polyphenols, may effectively reduce the incidence and severity of rheumatoid arthritis. Those mice who did develop RA had a less severe form of the disease.

If you decide to add green tea to your supplemental regimen, it couldn't be easier. Tea bags are found at grocery stores. Brew yourself a daily pot of green tea and reap the benefits.

Tart Cherry Juice

Some interesting laboratory research has found that anthocyanins, the chemicals that give tart cherries their color, may have more powerful anti-inflammatory effects than aspirin. A Johns Hopkins study found that anthocyanins from tart cherries were effective in treating inflammation-induced pain in rats. Evidence suggests that tart cherry anthocyanins may have a helpful role in reducing inflammatory pain.

If you can tolerate the acidic nature of tart cherry juice, you may consider adding this supplement to your arthritis treatment program.

The Least You Need to Know

- Dietary supplements are not regulated by the FDA.
- Botanicals are plants or plant parts that may have therapeutic medicinal value.
- Glucosamine and chondroitin may be of value in treating osteoarthritis.
- Little if any well-controlled scientific data exist to support many of the claims made by manufacturers and proponents of supplements and other dietary therapies.
- Super foods get a lot of hype, but it all boils down to eating a healthy, well-balanced diet.

Complementary Therapies: Practices and Procedures

In This Chapter

◆ Working with your body

◆ Holistic approaches

◆ Expanding your arthritis treatment options

◆ Avoiding scams

In a very real sense, complementary and alternative medicine (CAM) is the world's storehouse of medical lore, and today this storehouse is big business. American consumers spend as much as $14 billion a year on these medical treatments, looking for relief and in some cases, a cure. In this chapter, we'll take a look at the good, the not-so-good, and the downright dangerous.

Common Complementary Practices

Exploring complementary and alternative medicine (CAM) can take you on a journey through time and across cultures. Some types of complementary therapies strain the limits of credibility, others are close to being considered mainstream, and a few have even managed to cross the border and become naturalized citizens.

Acupuncture

Acupuncture is an ancient practice of the healing arts that originated in China over 2,000 years ago. In this traditional system, it is believed that energy, known as *qi*, flows through the body along specific pathways called meridians. If this energy is blocked, disease results. Inserting fine needles at specific points along the meridians was believed to unblock the *qi* so that energy could flow once again, restoring balance to the body.

> **Consultation**
>
> In today's Western medicine, researchers believe that acupuncture needles are responsible for releasing endorphins, the body's feel-good hormones, which promote pain relief by blocking pain signals from reaching the brain. Your physician may be trained in acupuncture.

An acupuncture treatment doesn't hurt, although there may be a slight tingling at the places where the needles are inserted. The acupuncturist may insert just a few needles or may use more, depending upon the type of treatment and the problem being addressed. The needles usually remain in place for 15 to 40 minutes, during which time you will rest quietly. After that, the acupuncturist removes the needles and you go on your way.

You may experience immediate relief from pain, although this may be initially short-lived. Additional treatments may increase the amount of time your pain is relieved. Research has found that acupuncture does indeed offer relief from pain:

♦ One recent study involved 10 arthritis patients with symmetric joint involvement. One of each patient's knees received an acupuncture treatment and the other received a sham treatment. Results found significant improvement in pain relief in the knee treated with real acupuncture compared with the knee treated with sham acupuncture. The acupuncture-treated knees remained pain-free for an average of one to three months compared to less than 10 hours for the sham acupuncture–treated knees.

♦ A 2004 study of the effects of acupuncture on nearly 600 people with osteoarthritis of the knee found that acupuncture relieved pain and improved function.

♦ Several 2006 studies of thousands of patients with chronic osteoarthritis pain compared acupuncture to conventional treatment (physical therapy and anti-inflammatory drugs). These studies showed positive results for acupuncture and suggested that acupuncture's benefits may be sustained for up to six months after treatment.

Risks involved are few. Needles should be used one time only and then disposed of, so there is no chance of transmitting disease from one patient to another. The American Academy of Medical Acupuncture's referral service lists more than 1,500 physicians with specialized training in acupuncture. Their website is www.medicalacupuncture.org.

Yoga

Yoga is a discipline uniting mind, body, and spirit. It comes to us from ancient India. Western practitioners have tended to use it primarily as a therapeutic form of exercise. Yoga's benefits go far beyond that of an exercise regimen, however, and as an adjunct to your arthritis treatment protocol, you might find its meditative aspects of considerable benefit.

The physical practice of yoga is often called hatha yoga. It can increase your strength, endurance, and balance and improve your postural alignment. The three components to most Western yoga classes are poses (*asanas*), breathing practices (*pranayama*), and relaxation. Meditation and chanting may also be part of the class.

Beginner and gentle yoga classes will not ask you to turn yourself into a pretzel or to assume uncomfortable poses. You start slowly and build flexibility and strength. You are not in competition with anyone else in the class and should not go beyond your comfort zone. You'll wear comfortable clothing that is neither too loose nor too tight. It's traditional to practice yoga barefoot.

Beginning *asanas* are generally simple standing and seated poses. Their purpose is to increase awareness of the body and its relationship to space. If your arthritis makes it difficult to sit cross-legged, you can sit in a chair or use a chair or another prop to support you. Poses can be modified for your comfort and still be beneficial.

Breathing is part of yoga. You will inhale for one direction of a pose, for example, and exhale for another direction of the pose. You may also hold a pose for a specific number of breaths.

Consultation

Studies on the benefits of yoga on osteoarthritis and rheumatoid arthritis are currently underway. The Johns Hopkins Arthritis Center (www.hopkins-arthritis.org) provides excellent information on practicing yoga if you have arthritis.

Yoga classes generally end with a period of relaxation, lasting from 1 to 15 minutes. You'll usually do this while lying on your back with your eyes closed. This is done to achieve the stress-relieving benefits of your poses and to promote a sense of well-being and peace. Many beginning yoga students think of this relaxation period as a reward for enduring the session! The purpose, however, is to prepare you for the meditative aspects to follow.

If you decide to give yoga a try, your local hospital, community center, senior center, or YMCA is likely to have information on yoga classes. Yoga Alliance is the worldwide accrediting body for yoga instructors. Their website is www.yogaalliance.org.

Chiropractic

Chiropractic is a healing discipline created by Daniel David Palmer in 1895. Palmer was an Iowa grocer, not a physician, but he wanted to find a method of curing disease that didn't involve drugs. Today most practitioners use the Palmer Method, named after the founder of chiropractic.

def•i•ni•tion

The word **chiropractic** means "done by hand." The founder of chiropractic, Daniel David Palmer, studied the human spine and applied the ancient practice of manipulation to the spine as a means of healing.

Until 1978, the traditional medical establishment didn't recognize chiropractic as a legitimate form of therapeutic treatment. This was primarily the result of a prevailing belief among many chiropractors that chiropractic could cure any disease—including cancer. When this position changed, the AMA accepted the use of chiropractic for treating some musculo-skeletal disorders.

Chiropractors treat patients using joint manipulation or adjustments. They may use chiropractic to treat the cycle of pain and loss of mobility that comes with arthritis. A study published in the *Annals of Internal Medicine* found that 63 percent of people who visited a rheumatologist for osteoarthritis, rheumatoid arthritis, or fibromyalgia also sought some form of complementary and alternative medicine. Chiropractic was the most commonly used form of CAM.

Chiropractic is not recommended for patients with rheumatoid arthritis, severe osteo-porosis, malignant or inflammatory spine conditions, or recent fractures or disloca-tions. It is also not recommended for people who are on blood-thinning medications. The most serious risks of chiropractic are stroke and spinal cord injury after manipu-lation of the neck. These are rare.

Doctors of Chiropractic (D.C.s) are not medical doctors (M.D.s). To earn a D.C. requires a minimum of two years of college and four years in a school of chiropractic. Their professional association is the American Chiropractic Association and their website is www.amerchiro.org.

Check with your primary-care physician or rheumatologist for a referral.

Massage Therapy

Massage has existed in one form or another ever since someone rubbed a sore arm or someone else's sore back. This probably goes back to the beginning of time.

Massage has a great deal to recommend it. It can relieve stress and anxiety, muscle tension, fatigue, and pain. Massage uses a variety of strokes, kneading, and tapping to move muscles and soft tissue. It can invigorate you and calm you at the same time.

Straight Talk

Hippocrates, the father of medicine, advised that doctors should be experienced in "rubbing that can bind a joint that is loose and loosen a joint that is too hard."

Massage therapy has become big business, with over a quarter of a million massage therapists practicing in the United States. Nearly one fifth of Americans are estimated to get at least one professional massage each year. Many of these are seeking relief from arthritis. There are several different types of therapeutic massage, including Swedish massage, deep tissue massage, myofascial release, trigger point therapy, acupressure, shiatsu, and reflexology.

Massage sessions usually last from 60 to 90 minutes. The cost may vary considerably, although if your physician writes a prescription for you, your health insurance may cover the cost of treatment. The professional association for massage therapists is the American Massage Therapy Association (AMTA). Their website is www.amtamassage.org.

Other Practices and Procedures

Acupuncture, chiropractic, and yoga have moved into mainstream American society, but not mainstream medicine for the most part. Other practices and procedures haven't done either. This may be because they haven't been sufficiently studied to prove their benefits—or because they have been and the benefit just wasn't there.

Some of these may be helpful, some may be harmless, and a few have the potential for causing serious damage.

Precautions _____

Many of the studies of complementary therapies are not controlled studies. That means they are not conducted according to the rigorous standards required of true scientific research. Couple that with the placebo effect, which ranges from 25 to 30 percent in most arthritis studies, and you'll realize you should be suspicious of extravagant claims.

Ayurveda

Ayurveda originated in India more than 5,000 years ago. It's a holistic approach to treating illness that specifically addresses arthritis. It is based on the belief that everything is composed of five elements: air, water, fire, earth, and ether (space).

According to Ayurveda, arthritis is caused by an excess of _ama_ (a sticky by-product of digestion) and a lack of _agni_ (digestive fire). Poor digestion may be the culprit, along with a weakened colon that accumulates undigested food and waste materials. This leads to toxins that can reach the joints.

Ayurveda considers three types of arthritis:

 ◆ _Vata_—joints crack, pop, become dry, and are not swollen.

 ◆ _Pitta_—joints are inflamed, swollen, painful, red, and hot to the touch.

 ◆ _Kapha_—joints are stiff, swollen, cold, and clammy, and movement relieves the pain

The belief is that your body is out of balance, and once balance is restored (by eliminating toxins) your symptoms will go away. Treatment techniques used for arthritis include healthy diet and lifestyle changes, ayurvedic herbal remedies and supplements, exercise, spiritual practices, yoga, massage, meditation, and gemstone therapy with "hot" gems such as rubies and garnets.

Finding an ayurvedic practitioner in the United States may be difficult. There are currently no standards for certification, and most practitioners have been trained in India.

The healthy lifestyle changes, yoga, massage, and other therapies are generally considered safe, although the use of herbs and the procedures for detoxing may be extremely dangerous. Read the section "Does Detoxing Help?" later in the chapter, and be sure to talk it over with your doctor before trying any detox program.

The Alexander Technique

Your mother was right when she told you to stand up straight! Body awareness can make a great deal of difference in how you feel and how you experience the symptoms of arthritis. If your posture is poor, if your muscles are tense, and if your movements are stiff, you're going to hurt. That's the thinking behind the Alexander Technique, developed at the end of the nineteenth century by an Australian actor, F. Matthias Alexander, who wanted to improve his voice.

Practitioners of the Alexander Technique call themselves teachers and see their role as helping you relearn proper body movements. How you use or abuse your body determines how well your joints hold up. Someone who treads heavily as she walks, for example, is moving too heavily, forcefully, and quickly. The muscles can't contract in time to provide cushioning for the joints, and the person may develop knee osteoarthritis as a result.

The first step in the Alexander Technique is becoming aware of these harmful movements. Then you learn better ways to move. The teacher cues the client through a series of light touches and directed movements.

The Alexander Technique has some similarities to physical therapy. Learning how to use your body effectively and efficiently can reduce pain and stiffness and increase your range of motion.

There are no adverse side effects reported with practicing the Alexander Technique, although finding a teacher may be a challenge. Their website is www.alexandertechnique.com.

Aromatherapy

Aromatherapy uses scented essential oils to promote healing. These oils can be inhaled or used during a massage or while bathing. These oils are very concentrated and are diluted in a carrier oil, so as not to irritate the skin. Unless you are allergic to a specific plant from which an essential oil is derived, aromatherapy is quite safe and also quite pleasant.

Aromatherapy is not a treatment for arthritis, but it can relieve stress and promote peace of mind, which may decrease the perception of pain. Numerous essential oils are recommended for arthritis:

- Lavender
- Juniper
- Thyme
- Rosemary
- Eucalyptus
- Chamomile
- Ginger
- Lemon
- Black pepper
- Camphor

No well-controlled scientific research studies have been conducted on the benefits of aromatherapy for arthritis. A recent, small, informal study of patients with knee OA at Tokyo Metropolitan Police Hospital found that more than 75 percent of patients who massaged lavender and rosemary camphor oil into their knees in the morning and at night over a two-week period experienced pain relief.

It could be that the gentle massaging caused the pain relief, or it may be that the pleasant aromas promoted a general feeling of well-being and activated the placebo response.

Aromatherapy is relatively inexpensive and may help you manage stress and relieve anxiety and fatigue—contributors to arthritis pain.

Does Detoxing Help?

Proponents of detoxing to treat arthritis believe that the symptoms of pain and inflammation are caused by the presence of toxins in the joints. Removing these toxins solves the problem. The process of detoxing can involve fasting (using juice or fruit), colon cleansing, or dietary supplements of fiber and certain herbs.

Since toxins are supposed to accumulate in the body as a result of breathing polluted air, smoking, or unhealthy diets, detoxing to treat rheumatoid arthritis is supposed to work by cleansing the bowels, kidneys, lungs, liver, and blood of these toxins. As a result, the immune system is supposed to be strengthened.

Recommendations for performing a colon cleanse include modifying your diet to increase your consumption of leafy green vegetables while decreasing your consumption of dairy, red meat, and other "mucus-producing" foods.

Detoxing advocates refer to an event called a "healing crisis" that may be experienced on the third or fourth day of the cleansing regimen. This is said to include symptoms such as sore throat, headache, lightheadedness, bad breath, and pimples. This is felt a normal indication that toxins are beginning to leave your body. Having a bowel movement may relieve these symptoms.

Definitely consult your physician before embarking on a detoxing regimen. Overly aggressive cleansing or detoxing can be dangerous or even life-threatening.

Homeopathy

Homeopathy was developed by a German physician in the late eighteenth century. Its name means "similar suffering," and it operates on the principle that "like cures like." If your joints are hot, swollen, and tender, for example, the homeopath may use apis, which is made from bee stings, to cause more of the same.

Materials used in homeopathy include highly diluted doses of minerals, plants, and herbs. One criticism of homeopathy is that the remedies used are in extremely diluted form. Use of these remedies can cause an "aggravation," which is a temporary flare-up of your symptoms. This is supposed to be a sign that the treatment is working.

def•i•ni•tion

Homeopathy is an alternative medicine practice operating on the principle that "like cures like."

Homeopathic remedies are available in health food stores and in pharmacies. Homeopathy is not a regulated medical profession, so there are risks to consulting a homeopath. Licensed medical doctors may also use certain homeopathic treatments.

A recent English study conducted at the Royal London Homoeopathic Hospital looked at the effects of homeopathy on 112 patients with rheumatoid arthritis. They found no evidence that active homeopathy improved the symptoms of RA in those patients.

If you are considering homeopathy as a supplement to your arthritis treatment, consult your rheumatologist before you begin.

Prolotherapy

Prolotherapy adopts the homeopathic principle of "like cures like." The term prolotherapy was coined in 1956 by the procedure's inventor, George S. Hackett, M.D., reflecting his belief that a *proliferation* of ligament and tendon tissue was necessary for joint health.

If a joint is inflamed, a sugar water or enzyme solution is injected into ligaments and tendons to temporarily increase the inflammation. This should spur the body into action, increasing the blood flow that carries nutrients to the area and creating new collagen, which then matures and shrinks, tightening the ligaments and making them stronger.

A study involving 27 patients with osteoarthritis in the finger joints was conducted at the University of Kansas Medical Center. Results indicated that prolotherapy resulted in significantly improved finger movement and range of motion. The study appeared in the August 1, 2000, issue of *The Journal of Alternative and Complementary Medicine*.

Prolotherapists claim that treating ligament and tendon problems with prolotherapy early on will prevent later development of osteoarthritis. They recommend prolotherapy especially for preventing knee OA. The average number of treatments recommended by prolotherapists is four to six, although sometimes ten or more may be required to achieve good results.

Definitely consult your rheumatologist before considering prolotherapy.

Magnetic Devices

Using magnets to treat arthritis may seem to be something out of weird science, but magnet therapy is said to promote faster healing and relieve pain.

Small magnetic discs are positioned over the painful area of the body and held in place with tape. According to the Mayo Clinic, the magnets used for therapy are 10 times stronger than a typical refrigerator magnet. The theory behind the therapy is that the magnet provides a continuous magnetic field that is supposed to relieve pain.

Precautions

Manufacturers of medical devices—including magnets intended for medical use—must be cleared by the FDA before they can marketed. To date, the FDA has not yet given this clearance.

Magnets used for therapy come in different strengths and sizes. If pain is slight, they may be left in place for just a few minutes; if pain is severe, they may remain in place for up to several days. You can wear your magnet as a bracelet or even buy a mattress pad equipped with magnets to give yourself a restful, magnetized night's rest!

Do they work? A 1997 study conducted at Baylor College of Medicine found that magnet therapy provided significant relief to patients with post-polio pain. Researchers are now interested in seeing if magnets may also help treat arthritis pain. The National Institutes of Health (NIH) is sponsoring this research. But currently no research supports the use of magnets to treat arthritis.

Magnet users claim that this therapy really does work. You can spend anywhere from a few dollars to several thousand dollars on magnets for therapy. Magnet therapy is generally considered to be safe, although pregnant women, people with pacemakers, and people with cancer should not try it.

Low-Level Laser Therapy

Low-level laser therapy (LLLT) has been around for about 10 years as a treatment for rheumatoid arthritis. It's a non-invasive procedure, which means it doesn't involve surgery. LLLT is used mainly on the hands, two to three times a week for three to four weeks. It uses a light source that's believed to generate photochemical reactions within the body's cells and to decrease pain and swelling.

A 2000 study involving 112 people treated with a four-week course of LLLT and 92 in placebo groups found that LLLT provided pain relief as well as improvements in morning stiffness and in flexibility of the palm. There was no evidence that the treatment was harmful in any way, and no one experienced any negative side effects.

Another 2000 study looked at LLLT for treating both RA and OA. Researchers found significant benefit for RA patients, but not for OA patients. Results were reported in the *Journal of Rheumatology.*

LLLT may be worth considering for short-term relief of RA symptoms, but it doesn't appear to have long-lasting benefits.

Hydrotherapy

"Taking the waters" is an ancient form of therapy for soothing the aches and pains of arthritis. The word hydrotherapy means using water for therapeutic purposes. At the very least, it's relaxing and stress-relieving, which can interrupt the pain cycle.

In the nineteenth century, mineral springs were in their heyday, and many communities in the United States grew up around them. Water saturated with calcium, potassium, iron, and sulfur (with its unmistakable aroma) bubbled up through rocks from the depths of the earth and spilled into pools, where bathers soaked and hoped to heal their aches and pains.

Straight Talk _____

Is it the mineral waters? No. The same renewal of life would have resulted had they sojourned anywhere amid pure air, beautiful scenery, and cheerful society.
—George E. Walton, M.D., *The Mineral Springs of the United States and Canada,* 1873

Many people report getting relief from hydrotherapy. Since mineral springs are often located at resorts that may be some distance from where you live, the vacation atmosphere likely also contributes to your heightened sense of well-being.

Copper Bracelets

Wearing a copper bracelet is an old folk remedy for arthritis that may go back as far as the ancient Greeks. A few studies involving animals have found that copper supplements taken orally might slow the progression of joint and tissue damage associated with arthritis. One human study done in the 1970s found that copper bracelets were more effective than a placebo.

Copper may have both an antioxidant and a pro-oxidant effect on the body. The antioxidant effect might have some limited effect on arthritis symptoms, but the prooxidant effect might cancel it out. You might get more benefit from a quarter cup of fresh blueberries. At any rate, unless you are allergic to copper, wearing a copper bracelet shouldn't cause you any harm.

Avoiding Quackery

"What have I got to lose? It couldn't hurt, could it?" When you're living with chronic pain, you're ready to try almost anything for the chance of relief. The answers to those questions are "Maybe nothing, maybe quite a bit" and "Maybe yes, maybe no." There really *are* differences among the various types of complementary and alternative medicine. Some are quite effective and some appear to be bogus.

In this chapter we've taken a look at some of the more popular practices associated with complementary and alternative medicine, and you've seen the research regarding their effectiveness. But what happens when a new product or procedure comes on the market? You need to know how to separate the real thing from the snake oil. Fortunately, here's where common sense will give you the upper hand. Some shifty marketing techniques recur repeatedly; here are some phrases that should make you suspicious …

- Act now! Offer ends soon!

- The new miracle cure the medical establishment doesn't want you to know about!

- Our (insert procedure) will cure your arthritis in one pain-free treatment or your money back!

- No drugs! Instant relief!

- All-natural (product or treatment)!

- Thousands of satisfied customers!

- No side effects ever!

- Overnight cure for all types of arthritis!

- Secret formula to cure arthritis discovered!

The goal of this kind of advertising is to get you excited—that's the reason for all the exclamation points—so that you'll suspend your common sense and give the product or treatment the benefit of the doubt.

Human nature loves a conspiracy, and the medical establishment has taken a fair number of hits. The truth is that at the present time there is no cure for arthritis, but when there is, your rheumatologist will be the first one to make sure you get it.

It's easy to visualize the medical establishment as some sort of corporate entity when you encounter the sensational ads and commercials, but it's actually made up of your family physician, the nurse who tends to you after surgery, the psychologist who helps you through the dark hours, and countless other individuals who have chosen careers in the service of others and the pursuit of health and wellness.

So look carefully and with a critical eye when you see something that seems too good to be true. Most likely, it is.

Get referrals for CAM procedures. Your physician can recommend a chiropractor, massage therapist, yoga class, or any other treatment that may benefit you and will not harm you. Legitimate CAM practitioners will be licensed by their state boards and will be members of their professional associations. Relying solely on testimonials from friends and acquaintances can be risky. Everyone's arthritis is different.

So do your homework and ask questions. Become an informed consumer of health products and services. You'll save money and enjoy improved health as a result.

The Least You Need to Know

- ◆ Complementary therapies are supplements, not replacements for your arthritis treatment.

- ◆ Always get a referral from your rheumatologist for any CAM procedure or product.

- ◆ CAM can expand your options for arthritis treatment.

- ◆ Be suspicious of products and services that seem too good to be true.

Part 4

Living with Arthritis

Arthritis doesn't just affect your joints. It affects every aspect of your life, from the time you rise and struggle to brew a pot of coffee to the time you retire and find you can't sleep because of the pain and discomfort. There are ways to manage arthritis and make life worth living again. Arthritis doesn't have to control you. In Part 4, you'll learn strategies to gain the upper hand against arthritis.

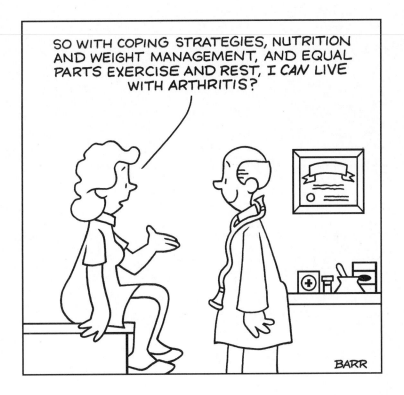

SO WITH COPING STRATEGIES, NUTRITION AND WEIGHT MANAGEMENT, AND EQUAL PARTS EXERCISE AND REST, I *CAN* LIVE WITH ARTHRITIS?

BARR

Chapter 13

Coping with Chronic Disease

In This Chapter

- Taking charge of your life
- Rethinking old patterns
- Looking beyond beauty
- Stress management
- Coping strategies
- How arthritis impacts sexuality

A chronic medical condition does much more than impact your physical health. It affects your emotional and spiritual health as well, and impacts the lives of your family, friends, and all those who care about you. Coming to terms with arthritis doesn't mean giving up. It does mean, however, that you accept the reality of arthritis and still choose to live your life on your own terms. Tackling each problem as it arises will increase your ability to cope in the long run. In this chapter, we'll cover some of these problems and look for solutions.

Coming to Terms

Before you can cope with a chronic illness, such as arthritis, you first need to come to terms with it. What does that mean? It means acceptance, but acceptance doesn't mean giving in and giving up. It does mean that you recognize your life is going to take a different tack and you understand that you're going to have to make some changes. You're going to learn to cope. To *cope* literally means to slash or to strike a blow, to fight or contend with successfully or on equal terms. When you learn to cope with arthritis, you're setting yourself up to be the victor!

Terminology about illness has changed in recent years, and the change has been so subtle that you're probably not aware of it. The change, however, has been both significant and positive. For example, we no longer say someone is *confined* to a wheelchair, but rather that she is *assisted* by a wheelchair. It's a very big difference. Being assisted is rich in connotations and conveys the idea of forward motion, of living life, and of having control.

Other terms have changed as well, but they all now put the emphasis on the person, not the disease or the medical condition. We've always done this to some extent. You've never considered someone with heart disease to *be* heart disease or someone with cancer to *be* cancer. That would be nonsense.

Somehow this intelligent approach didn't translate across the board, though, so we referred to people with deafness as *deaf* or people with blindness as *blind*. It's not a small distinction.

If you say, "Jim is deaf," you're actually doing some math. You're making an equation:

 ◆ Jim = deaf

 ◆ Sally = blind

 ◆ Jorge = speech impediment

> **Straight Talk**
>
> You learn to live with it. You don't like it, but it is a fact of life.
>
> —Jerry, age 58, diagnosed with osteoarthritis

You're nitpicking, you might be saying, but take a closer look. When your words equate someone with a disease or a condition—when you actually say that that person *is* that condition, you create unintended consequences. You consciously or unconsciously take that person's abilities down a notch. By putting the person first, you're putting the medical condition in its proper place. It's a factor, to be sure, but it's not the factor that determines a person's worth.

The same holds true for arthritis. You aren't arthritis; rather, you're a person with arthritis. Your medical condition has not changed who you are. It may have changed what you can do or how you do it, but it doesn't control your life, unless you let it.

Bottom line? Come to terms with arthritis and then move forward.

Your first priority, of course, is getting a handle on your symptoms. You're taking your prescribed medications, exercising, resting when you need to, and using whatever assistive devices make your life easier. What's next? Living your life.

Chronic Pain and Depression

Pain is one of the hallmark symptoms of arthritis, and, simply put, chronic pain wears you down. It erodes your overall outlook on life and turns daily tasks into monumental chores. You become irritable and short-tempered. You become less active because movement hurts, but restricted movement can cause isolation and frustration at not being connected to the world outside your pain.

How common is depression in people with chronic pain? Depression has been found to be the single most important variable associated with persistent chronic pain. In one analysis of 1,016 HMO members, people with three or more pain issues were 12 percent more likely to experience the symptoms of depression than those without pain issues or those with only one pain complaint. If your pain results in loss of independence or mobility, your risk of depression is significantly increased.

Depression has been defined as "anger turned inward." It's a good description. You may be angry at your body for what you perceive as a betrayal. It can help to think of your body as a valiant soldier fighting the good fight against pain and the other symptoms of arthritis. Don't fall into the trap of seeing your body as either the villain or the victim. Talk to your physician about how best to help your body attack the pain.

Precautions

The risk for depression extends beyond the person experiencing chronic pain. Studies of families of people with chronic pain have found that, compared to the general population, people with chronic pain had more first-degree relatives with depression and depressive disorders.

Depression can make everything that's bad worse. Pain hurts more. What may have been difficult before now seems impossible. You may find yourself feeling overwhelmed. If your depression is mild, you may not even realize you have it. Learn to recognize the symptoms of depression:

- Feeling down or blue for at least two weeks

- Difficulty falling or staying asleep

- Sleeping much less or much more than usual

- Difficulty concentrating

- Feeling helpless and that your life is hopeless

- Feeling that things you used to enjoy are now too much trouble and not worth the effort

- Loss of energy

- Thoughts of suicide

Depression can be a stand-alone medical condition, a symptom of another condition (such as hypothyroidism), or a side effect of certain medications. Regardless of the cause, depression can be treated. If you find your symptoms are interfering with your life and your ability to work, and if they last longer than two weeks, make an appointment with your doctor and get some help. If you feel overwhelmed and are actually thinking of ending your life, make a phone call. Call 1-800-SUICIDE and talk to someone who cares. Life is precious.

Self-Esteem Issues

How we feel about ourselves has a great deal to do with how we feel physically. When we're feeling on top of the world, we're confident, self-assured, and able to take on anything that gets thrown at us. Unfortunately, the opposite is also true. When we're not feeling well, our self-image suffers and we're likely to be less confident in our abilities. It's just human nature.

Especially if your form of arthritis results in noticeable physical changes, such as swollen knuckles or a limp, you may think everyone is staring at you and feeling sorry for you. But the truth may be something quite different from your perceptions.

Everyone has limitations and physical difficulties of one sort or another. That person you see looking at you might be thinking how confident you are to not let a physical problem stop you from living your life, and may wish that she had some of that confidence to help her cope with her own problems.

When you're not feeling good about yourself, those views have a tendency to spread and color your perceptions about the world in general. Negative thoughts crowd out positive ones. You think you should be able to control your own body, and you're frustrated that you can't. So often control is an illusion—there's really very little in life that we have control over—but there *is* one thing you can control, and that's your response to whatever difficulties you're facing.

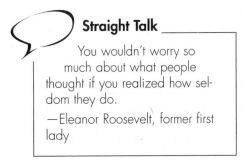

Straight Talk

You wouldn't worry so much about what people thought if you realized how seldom they do.

—Eleanor Roosevelt, former first lady

Appearance Concerns

It's only natural to want to look your best. That doesn't mean you have to have movie-star looks, but it does mean that you take pride in your personal appearance. Why? It shows the world that you know who you are, that you're confident in your abilities, and that you're prepared to meet whatever challenges come your way. It conveys the message that you're at the top of your game. That's quite a statement to make to the world simply on the basis of good grooming and tasteful attire.

Throughout history and across cultures, certain standards of physical beauty prevailed. These standards, however, change over time. For example, in earlier days, being overweight meant that you were wealthy—you could afford to buy whatever you wanted. Today, the opposite is true. Thin is in. Sometimes too thin, judging by the number of anorexic celebrities flocking to counseling and rehab programs.

Symmetry is also considered important. People whose faces are symmetrical are perceived as more handsome or beautiful than those whose faces are off-kilter. Plato tried his hand at deconstructing beauty and determined that the width of the ideal face should be two thirds of its length, and that the nose should not be any longer than the distance between the eyes.

So, what does this mean for the vast majority of the world's population who don't fit into these tight little categories? It means that we must find our self-worth in more substantial ways. There really is no perfect body or perfect face. And even if there were, Father Time marches on anyway. Cultivate your interests, develop your skills, and focus on what matters.

Some forms of arthritis can be disabling. If rheumatoid arthritis isn't well controlled, for example, your joints may become deformed, particularly the joints in your hands and feet. If this happens, you may become self-conscious about your appearance and may avoid situations where you feel as if you are on display.

The March 2007 issue of *Arthritis Care and Research* dealt with the dynamics of physical appearance concerns and depression and anxiety in people who were newly diagnosed and those who were dealing with chronic rheumatoid arthritis and lupus.

Investigators used surveys to determine how people viewed various aspects of their health, their levels of psychological distress, and the coping skills they used in daily life. What they found was that all groups showed greater psychological distress than people in the general population who had not been diagnosed with arthritis.

Among those with lupus, 53 percent reported feeling that the disease made them unattractive, while 30 percent of those with chronic rheumatoid arthritis and 34 percent of those newly diagnosed with rheumatoid arthritis had these concerns.

How to address these issues? First, acknowledge them. Validating your concerns is the first step. It's important to be sure you are following your treatment program and checking with your rheumatologist if your symptoms are concerning you. If you feel that your arthritis is affecting your self-image, a mental health professional can help you process these feelings and make some changes that can alter your perspective. Some simple strategies can help you get over this hurdle and emerge a more self-confident person:

- ◆ Each morning, look at yourself in the mirror. Then smile. Notice how your face lifts and your eyes light up. Even if you have to force it, make this part of your morning routine. You may think there's nothing to smile about, but smile anyway. Put on a happy expression and you'll set the tone for the entire day.

- ◆ Brush your teeth and comb your hair. Step in the shower and get the blood flowing throughout your body.

- ◆ Get dressed. Be comfortable but not sloppy. How you dress will affect everything from your posture to your attitude.

- ◆ Be grateful for your body that is working so hard to fight arthritis. Nourish it with a good breakfast. Start the day with good nutrition and you give your body fuel for the fight.

♦ Commit to exercise. Strengthen your muscles that support your joints. Become as fit as you can.

Remind yourself often of your worth. You have much to contribute, and arthritis hasn't taken that away from you. You may need to find different ways to make that contribution, but that will only make you stronger—and strength is beautiful.

Attitude Is Everything

Well, it may not be everything, but it's certainly important. It's easy to fall into the trap of feeling sorry for yourself and bemoaning the fact that life isn't fair. That's no breaking news, however. Life has never been fair, but you've got what it takes to rise above the ruts in the road. Adjust your attitude to positive and look for the humor in the ridiculous, and you'll find that you gradually feel better about yourself.

You are much more than joints and ligaments and cartilage and the various other components that make up your physical body. You have talents and gifts and qualities that make you uniquely you, and arthritis cannot take them away from you. Ever.

So, how to go about improving your self-image? Making a list is one way to start. Write down everything that's wrong with you. Don't stop until you can't think of another thing. Include even the smallest things you can dredge up. Then take a look at your list and see what you've got. Items toward the top will probably relate to your arthritis and are likely to include your physical symptoms. Items toward the end are likely to look like the results of a poor fishing expedition. Hangnails are a problem for you?

The next step is to make a list of all your positive traits. List everything that's right about you. Again, don't stop until you've totally run out of ideas. Include even the smallest items. When you look at your list, you'll likely notice that items toward the top relate to your character. For example, you're honest. You're thoughtful. You're kind to animals. You're also likely to notice that the items toward the bottom of your list are the ones associated with your physical characteristics. For example, you have a nicely shaped nose.

Finally, put your two lists together. They'll most likely be mirror images of each other, with your disabilities at the top and your negative character flaws at the bottom. Your list of positives is also likely to be longer than your list of negatives. Your task is to strike a balance and put things in perspective. Arthritis can be a devastating medical condition that sends you down for the count, or it can be a challenge that you take on and refuse to let get the better of you. It's all a matter of attitude.

Managing Stress

Uncertainty aggravates stress, and when you have a chronic medical condition you can't help but wonder about what the future holds. Stress builds. Without a positive outlet for that stress, your symptoms can worsen. It becomes a vicious cycle. You worry about your ability to continue functioning at work and then you worry about the financial difficulties that may result from this. You feel a loss of control.

Consultation

If you have rheumatoid arthritis, you may find that you experience a flare shortly after going through a stressful event. You may not be imagining the connection. Recently, immunologists have found that stress can affect your body's immune response. Reducing stress, then, is important.

Stress is a normal reaction to situations that require some type of action. Once you've acted, the stress goes away. Stress that results from a chronic medical condition builds. Not only does this affect you, but it also affects your family, friends, and work associates.

If you begin to feel overwhelmed by stress, it's wise to seek help from a mental health professional. Individual counseling, along with support groups, can make a world of difference in how you are able to cope with arthritis. You'll learn strategies for managing stress and ways to minimize its negative impact on your life.

Support groups come with another benefit, as well: shared humor. You can let your hair down with others who share your same fears and frustrations, and humor is a time-honored way of coping with them. Learn to laugh at the absurd and the ridiculous, and you'll find that arthritis loses its power to control you.

When you're overwhelmed with feelings of hopelessness, it can be empowering to realize that other people have also felt this way and have managed to overcome it. They'll share their coping strategies with you and, in turn, you'll find that you have helpful information to share with them.

Precautions

Alcohol can intensify the symptoms of depression, so limit your intake of alcohol to avoid making your situation worse.

If you aren't comfortable discussing your private issues in a group setting, then one-on-one professional counseling may be more appropriate for you. Your rheumatologist can refer you to a mental health professional.

Raising Your Expectations

It's one of those strange facts of life that you generally get what you expect you deserve. In some cases this works out fine, but in others the payoff is less than satisfactory. For example, some people believe that life just happens to them and they have no part in the process. Other people believe in becoming actively involved in their own lives and having some say in the matter.

People who fall into that first category are showing a mind-set that's called *learned helplessness*. They don't think there's a thing they can do to cope with chronic illness, so they don't cope at all. Of course, you know this isn't logical, since there's a great deal you can do to cope with arthritis.

People in the second category understand that chronic illness may put some limitations on their lives, but they work to find ways to adapt and to continue enjoying life. These people, and you are undoubtedly one of them, are showing behavior that's called *self-efficacy*. It's quite basic: what you believe will have a huge impact on how you feel.

Several research studies have examined how these two different mind-sets affected the lives of people with rheumatoid arthritis. Researchers found that learned helplessness was linked to higher levels of arthritis pain, depression, and disability, while self-efficacy was linked to reductions in pain, depression, and disease activity. A review of these studies appeared in the 1999 issue of *Rheumatic Disease Clinics of North America*.

Here's a list of thinking patterns to avoid:

- **Jumping to conclusions.** You're having a flare and think that this time it's permanent. It's never going away. The reality: You're having a flare. You'll slow down, rest, and take your medications, and since arthritis follows a fairly predictable pattern, the flare will subside over the next few days.

- **It's gotta be all or nothing.** If you can't do everything you ever did in the exact same way, then there's nothing you can do. Period. The reality: There are all kinds of adaptive devices available to help you do your work, assist you in getting dressed, and generally make your life easier.

- **Overgeneralizing.** You see one negative event as leading to a downward spiral of failure. You can't wash the windows anymore, so you figure you're worthless. You'll never be of any use again. The reality: You can hire someone to clean the windows. High school students are always looking for ways to make some spending money. While you're supervising the window washing, make a list of all the things you *can* still do. You'll probably still be working on that list after the windows are finished.

◆ **Mental filtering.** You focus on one negative aspect until it crowds out all the positives. You're fatigued, but the swelling, stiffness, and pain have significantly decreased. All you can think about is your fatigue, and you figure that means your arthritis is getting worse. The reality: You may be anemic and this can be treated. (Start by reading Chapter 15.)

◆ **Ignoring the positive.** If you ignore the positive, all that leaves is the negative. You wake up feeling rested but that doesn't matter. Your knee is stiff. The reality: Balance your perspective. Be thankful you've got some energy (because of your good night's rest) to cope with that bothersome knee.

Rheumatoid arthritis (RA) can be potentially disabling and disfiguring. However, your attitude and your outlook are more powerful than RA, and you can lead a productive and satisfying life even while you wait for the cure.

Gender Patterns

Women are more likely than men to use coping strategies to deal with arthritis pain. They're also better at lessening the emotional fallout of chronic pain. Those are the findings of a recent study sponsored by the National Institutes of Health (NIH) and conducted by researchers at Ohio University.

For the study, 48 men and 99 women diagnosed with either osteoarthritis or rheumatoid arthritis were asked to keep a daily log of their activities. Over a 30-day period, these study participants recorded how much pain they were feeling and how they responded to that pain. Researchers found that when women were experiencing pain, they used a variety of coping mechanisms, which included relaxation, distraction, and seeking emotional support from others.

While the women in the study reported having more joint pain than the men, their moods on the days after high pain levels weren't negatively impacted. The men had a different pattern. They reported that their moods were poor after these high-pain days. What's interesting about this study is that none of the women had had training in formal coping skills. They developed these on their own.

What researchers discovered may be linked to what our culture expects from men: Don't show your pain, keep your fears private, don't ever show weakness. These may have been necessary survival traits for our ancestors, but in today's world, their usefulness is limited. The researchers concluded that men may need to be taught coping skills to help them manage their arthritis pain.

Support from Your Spouse

It can be difficult to know how much someone else is hurting. In one study designed to measure a spouse's ability to detect his or her partner's pain, researchers looked at both sides of this issue. They videotaped 19 osteoarthritis patients doing daily activities, such as sitting, standing, and walking. Each patient then watched the videotape and graded the pain he or she felt during each act on a scale ranging from "no pain" to "pain as bad as it can be." Then the spouses watched the tape and used the same scale to assign a value to their partner's pain.

The results? Women were better at assessing their partners' pain than were men. Researchers found that while women were more perceptive about how their partners were feeling, they could benefit from special training in helping their partners deal more effectively with that pain.

Practical Tips

In addition to the emotional aspects of coping with chronic illness, there are the day-to-day tasks that must be done. Learning how to do these jobs while conserving your energy is an essential coping skill. Common sense is the common denominator.

It can be all too tempting to try to push yourself when you're feeling better. You overdo, but you pay the price. Use the two-hour rule to assess your pain: If you have pain that lasts for two hours or more after an activity or exercise, then you've done too much. Next time you're tempted to push your limits, remember what you're likely to experience afterward and make some adjustments.

If you learn the proper ways to bend, lift, reach, and stretch, you're less likely to strain your muscles and joints. Your physical therapist can teach you these methods.

Staying in one position for an extended period of time can cause your joints to stiffen up, so change your position frequently. Do some mild stretches and range of motion exercises to increase your flexibility and lessen pain and stiffness.

Consultation

Use your largest and strongest joints and muscles. When you lift or carry objects, use your arms instead of your hands, to avoid placing too much stress on one joint or one area of your body.

It's also important to learn how to balance periods of activity with periods of rest. Listen to what your body is telling you. If you're beginning to get tired, it's time to stop. If you stop early, you'll be able to start up again much sooner than you would if you pushed yourself just to get the job finished. Even when you're feeling good, remember to keep that rest/work balance in balance!

Some strategies that help in coping with arthritis make good sense in general. For example, conserve your energy by simplifying your tasks. Do some advance planning before you begin a task. Gather all the supplies you'll need, and you'll avoid having to stop and look for what you need. This saves both time and energy.

If an activity causes you joint pain, do some assessment. There are jar openers, reach extenders, zipper pulls, and large-handled utensils that take the strain off your joints. Your occupational therapist has catalogs with all kinds of products that can make your life simpler and less painful.

Finally, ask for help when you need it. You don't have to be the Lone Ranger. Everybody needs help at times, and that's what family and friends are for. There will be a time when they'll need you to help them out, so don't be afraid to ask for help when you need it. Other coping strategies include …

- Maintaining a healthy body weight. Being overweight puts extra stress on weight-bearing joints such as your back, hips, knees, and feet.

- Sitting, instead of standing, to do a job when you can.

- Respecting the pain. It's your body telling you something is wrong.

- Use a shoulder strap to carry a purse or computer bag instead of gripping the handle with your hand.

- Distributing weight to decrease the stress on any one joint. Lift with your palms rather than with your fingers. Carry heavy loads in your arms instead of with your hands.

Your local chapter of the Arthritis Foundation offers classes on self-help strategies, and it's worth your while to check them out. Arthritis self-help courses are designed for people of any age who have arthritis. They also are designed for family members and caregivers and for people who have risk factors for developing arthritis. It's a two-hour, six-week course, covering a wide variety of topics, including …

- The effects diet and exercise have on arthritis and osteoporosis.

- Cognitive pain management strategies.

- Effects of medication use.

- Recipes and nutrition guides appropriate for those with arthritis.

- Strategies for dealing with depression.

- Evaluation of new and alternative treatment options.

- How to work more effectively with health-care providers

- Fatigue and sleep loss stemming from arthritis

- How to increase exercise endurance and conserve energy

And an added benefit is connecting with others who share your concerns. It becomes a support group where you can exchange ideas and solve problems.

Sexuality and Arthritis

Sexuality is a broad topic, and arthritis can impact your sexuality in various ways. Fatigue, side effects of medications, painful joints, and a poor self-image can all contribute to diminished sexual activity. You can reclaim your love life, however, if you're open to making some changes. Your doctor can provide you with good information.

When arthritis involves your hips, knees, or spine, sexual intimacy can be more painful than pleasurable. This is the time to experiment with new positions that take pressure off affected joints; for example, both partners lie on their sides. Also, planning your romantic interludes can allow you to have time to take your pain medication and indulge in a warm shower to ease stiffness an hour or so before.

Changing the time of day you have sex can also make an important difference. If you are stiff and sore in the mornings, consider afternoons or early evenings instead.

Talk to your partner. If you simply find ways to avoid sex, your partner may feel that he or she is somehow to blame. Open and honest communication will prevent hurt feelings. You know what hurts and what gives you pleasure, but your partner cannot read your mind. Even if talking about sex is difficult for you, give it a try. This is one area of your life where communication is vital. And it gets easier with practice. Remember to let your partner know when something feels good, and it will be easier to say when something hurts.

Consultation

An added benefit of sex is that it causes your body to release endorphins, the body's own natural painkillers. It's a free prescription!

The Arthritis Foundation (see Appendix C) offers a pamphlet titled "Living and Loving: Information about Sexuality and Intimacy." The document includes diagrams of a variety of positions and techniques used by people with arthritis to make the most of their love lives.

The Least You Need to Know

- Your personal worth isn't determined by your medical condition—don't let arthritis define you.

- Your attitude can influence how you feel, so cultivate a positive perspective. Expect to live a rich, full life, and you will!

- Ask for help when you need it. Your family and friends are there for you.

- Don't ignore your sexuality—it's part of the good life.

14

Self-Help Strategies for Pain Management

In This Chapter

- ◆ Pain basics
- ◆ Gaining control of your pain
- ◆ The mind-body connection
- ◆ Proactive strategies
- ◆ Finding support

Pain can be acute or chronic, mild or severe, confined to one spot or felt throughout your body. Everyone feels pain differently. What may seem just an annoying ache to you may feel like agony to someone else. Everyone agrees, however, that chronic pain is one of the most difficult aspects of dealing with arthritis.

Arthritis pain can vary from day to day and even throughout the course of one day. In addition to its physical aspects, pain can create fallout in the emotional, psychological, social, and occupational parts of your life. In this chapter, we'll discuss self-help strategies to help you effectively manage pain and reduce its negative impact on your life.

What Causes Pain

The pain response is a complex system. When your joints become inflamed, pain-sensing neurons, or pain receptors, in the affected area send a message to your spinal cord, which relays it to your brain. Your brain processes the message and relays a response through those neurons back down your spinal cord, prompting you to act to relieve the source of the pain.

> **Consultation**
>
> Pain receptors are located throughout your body, with the main clusters associated with your skin, joint surfaces, the lining around the bone (called the periosteum), arterial walls, and areas within the skull. Your brain has no pain receptors at all and can't detect pain!

The mechanics are complicated, but the purpose of the message is simple. It's designed to get you to do something about the situation that's triggering that pain response. Your first message is "I hurt." Then you analyze: "Where do I hurt?" "Why do I hurt?" All this happens very quickly, but after you answer those two questions, you can begin to address the problem and do something about your pain. There are two kinds of pain: acute and chronic.

Acute Pain

Acute pain comes on fast, often as the result of an injury. It can be sharp, stabbing, or throbbing and gets your attention immediately. Headaches, cramps, and appendicitis fall into this category. First aid, emergency surgery, or aspirin, along with time, usually take care of the problem. "Time heals all wounds" probably derived from these kinds of acute situations.

Chronic Pain

Chronic pain is different from acute pain. This kind of pain hangs around long after an injury has healed, or it may be a symptom of disease. Pain that lasts longer than three months is considered to be chronic, although some experts consider pain chronic only if it lasts more than six months. Almost 66 million Americans deal with arthritis pain and about 43 million of them are coping with chronic pain.

Chronic arthritis pain is caused by a combination of factors, both physical and emotional. Inflammation and damage to the joint tissues are physical factors. Fatigue is as well, though it can be complicated by feelings of stress and depression. You'll read more about the insidious role of fatigue in Chapter 15. Depression can also cause increased pain. If you are feeling fatigued or depressed and you've lost interest in activities you used to enjoy, talk to your physician. Chronic illness can lead to depression, a medical condition that usually responds well to treatment.

Perceptions of Pain

How you perceive pain is to a great extent a product of your genetics. Researchers have discovered that a particular gene is responsible for regulating how your brain responds to pain. What this means for arthritis is that your experience of pain and discomfort is uniquely your own. This means that your treatment plan will also be unique to you. In addition to chronic fatigue and depression, other factors also play a role in determining how much the pain of arthritis will affect you. These *stressors* include …

- Stress.

- Previous experience with pain.

- Increased disease activity.

- Worry and anxiety.

- Focusing on the pain.

Stress is a normal part of living and it's a big contributor to how severely you feel pain. Stress itself is neither good nor bad—how you react to stress, however, determines its effects on your body. People dependent upon others for their care, such as children or the elderly, or those who lack a support system are more at risk for stress-related medical conditions.

def•i•ni•tion

In medical terms, a **stressor** is anything that upsets the balance of physical reactions in your body. Your reaction to stress is to a large extent a function of your personality, general health, physical strength, and psychological well-being.

Stress gears your body up for the fight-or-flight reaction and can be life-saving in dangerous situations. It's meant to come quickly, be acted upon quickly, and then leave just as quickly. Today, however, stress builds. You can't run away from the pressures of modern living, and the constant state of fight-or-flight preparedness takes a toll on your body as well as your mind.

Symptoms of stress? Your muscles get tight, your breathing becomes fast and shallow, your heart rate increases, and your blood pressure rises. Your body is preparing to face the enemy. In this case, however, the enemy is arthritis, and the body is not helping with these responses, but instead is increasing your perception of pain. Learning to manage stress is essential for managing arthritis.

Examine what increases your stress levels. If these stressors are of your own making, then some stress reduction is in order. If you're a last-minute kind of person, arthritis may be making that last minute overly painful and less productive than it once was. How to help this? Plan ahead! Break large tasks into smaller ones and get these out of the way as you feel able. Then at the last minute you won't have everything looming over your head.

Practicing avoidance is another technique for managing stress. This means avoiding people, places, or situations that raise your stress to uncomfortable levels. If you cannot totally eliminate these stressors, try to at least minimize your exposure to them.

Along with stress come worry and anxiety. These may be caused in part by increased disease activity. When you're experiencing a flare, it's only natural to be concerned. You may wonder if this time the flare will be more severe, last longer, or leave more damage in its wake. At these times it becomes difficult not to focus on your pain. You do have options, however, and developing a pain management plan is one of them.

A Pain Management Plan

Pain will occupy as big a part of your life as you're willing to give it. You may not be able to eliminate pain, but you can take positive action to limit its effects on your physical, mental, and emotional health. Since each type of arthritis can cause different kinds of pain, you'll first need to get a clear understanding of your pain and how it's impacting your life.

You can't ignore your pain, so it's best to find a way to control it and your response to it. One way to get started managing your pain is to begin recording your symptoms in order to get insight into your day-to-day pain.

Keeping a Pain Diary

It's been said that the worst diary is better than the best memory, and that certainly holds true when dealing with medical matters. Even if you've never kept a diary or a journal before, you'll find it's well worth trying it to help you get an accurate perspective on your symptoms. For the next two weeks, make the commitment to document your symptoms.

From One to Ten

Your pain will vary in intensity during the course of the day. It may be more severe upon waking, after sitting for a while or after periods of inactivity, when you retire for the night, or when you're engaged in physical activity. Whenever you experience pain, give your pain a number from 1 to 10 (1 being mild and 10 being excruciating) and write that number down, along with the time of day and what you were doing when you felt the pain. If you can identify triggers for your pain, you'll be well on your way to managing it. Be faithful to your diary and you'll be rewarded with valuable information.

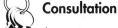

Consultation

Invest in a small notebook, rather than relying on loose sheets of paper that are easily misplaced or thrown away. A little spiral notebook fits easily in a pocket or purse, and you'll be more inclined to jot down symptoms if your paper is handy.

If you are taking medication for your arthritis, keep it in mind as you keep your pain diary. Is your medication effective in managing your pain? Ask yourself …

◆ Does your pain return before it's time for the next dose?

◆ How long does it take to get relief after you've taken your medication?

Here's what a sample journal page might look like.

7:00 A.M. Left knee very stiff and sore upon waking. Pain in knee woke me up twice during the night. (8 on the scale)

7:30 A.M. Took prescription medication.

8:45 A.M. Knee felt much better. (4)

12:30 P.M. Severe knee pain. Throbbing. (9)

2:00 P.M. Took prescription medication.

3:00 P.M. Pain much better. (4)

Your task here is not to diagnose. It's just to observe and record. As you can see, your notes don't have to be elaborate. Just write down what you are feeling.

Putting the Plan in Motion

Two weeks is a good length of time to track your pain. It's long enough to allow for fluctuations, variations, and patterns to become evident. After you've collected your data, take your diary to your next rheumatology appointment and discuss your findings with your doctor. With this information, you and your rheumatologist can develop a pain management plan especially designed to help you deal with your type of arthritis. That plan is likely to include medications, physical therapy, exercise, and perhaps surgery. And there is one more course of action that can be an effective addition to these treatments: self-help strategies.

Their primary benefits? They're cost-effective—they're free. They require no special equipment, you can use them almost anywhere, you don't need to make an appointment, and most important of all—they work.

Coping with chronic disease can make you feel powerless. Developing a plan to manage that disease, however, is proactive and empowering and will reduce the grip arthritis has on you. Here's a look at some worthwhile additions to your pain management program. The mind-body connection is very real and you can use it to get maximum pain relief.

As you begin to take control of your pain, it's helpful to remember that establishing a new habit takes about three weeks. You have to unlearn the old habit and replace it with the new one. This takes time, and you may be tempted to give up, but persevere. It's well worth the time and the effort.

Reframing Your Thinking Patterns

How you look at something is a function of your personality. And yes, it's true that optimistic types have an easier time with this part of pain management. However, even if you're the kind of person who doesn't consider whether the glass is half full or half empty because you notice that it's chipped, there is hope.

It's all about power and control. When you are in pain and feeling miserable because of it, then arthritis has the power and it also has control over how you react to the pain. Positive thinking reverses this scenario and reinvests the power in you.

If pain is the center of your life, then pain will color and affect everything you say, feel, think, and do. To get relief from your pain, it's essential to change your focus. In fact, taking your mind off your pain is the first step in managing that pain.

Negatives into Positives

It's easy to let negative thoughts crowd into your mind. The trick is to recognize them when they show up and learn strategies for turning them around. The next time your mind latches onto a negative, such as, "I'm always in pain; I'll never feel any better," turn the thought around: "I'm going to keep at my exercise program, take my medications, and do everything I can to feel better. Arthritis does not control my life." Repeating this to yourself as often as necessary will eventually change your negative thought pattern into a more positive—and more productive one.

Positive self-talk is positive thinking's first cousin. With positive self-talk you become your own advocate. You don't wait for the negatives to intrude, but instead you take the upper hand right away. "I'm going to exercise today, so I'll have a good appetite and will sleep better tonight." Keep that focus throughout the day and you'll feel better.

In a 2005 study, researchers confirmed that if you expect your pain to be less severe, you will actually perceive less pain. In fact, they found about a 28 percent decrease in how people perceived pain, and that equated to relief obtained with a shot of morphine. The study was reported in the September 2005 online edition of the *Proceedings of the National Academy of Sciences*.

> **Straight Talk**
>
> Even on my worst days, when I couldn't hold my trowel, I'd walk out into my garden and ignore the weeds. I'd smell the roses and their fragrance helped get me through.
>
> —Julie, age 56, diagnosed with rheumatoid arthritis at 40

Distraction

You have the ability to decide what will occupy your thoughts. It's difficult to keep track of two things at once, something we've all experienced on busy days when there seem to be a hundred tasks that need doing. If you find that pain is constantly on your mind, distract yourself. Give your mind something else to think about. Not sure how to begin? If you've been sitting down, get up!

Even if it hurts, getting moving is good for you. Sometimes pain is just your body telling you that you've been doing something for too long. Changing your position or changing your activity may be all you need to do. Need some suggestions?

- ◆ Sing

- ◆ Meditate

- ◆ Go for a walk

- ◆ Visit a friend

- ◆ Watch a good movie

- ◆ Spend time on a hobby

The possibilities are endless. What gives you joy?

Relaxation Techniques

When you're dealing with arthritis, your muscles are working hard to support your swollen or inflamed joints. Pain causes those muscles to tense up. Muscle tension causes more pain, and then you're stuck in a vicious cycle. It's time to relax and let your muscles get a rest. There are several kinds of relaxation strategies you can use to help your body get some relief.

Precautions

Your bedroom should be a place exclusively reserved for sleep and sex. Your mind makes powerful associations, and if your bedroom does double duty as a home office, you're going to have difficulty relaxing!

Progressive relaxation is a technique you can do at night, as you lie in bed ready to go to sleep. You think about each part of your body and invite it to relax. You start at your toes, then work your way up to your legs, your trunk, your arms, your hands, and, finally, your head. As you become aware of your joints, especially your painful ones, let your mind gently scan them and encourage them to relax. No one is watching and no one can hear your thoughts, so give it a try! You may find this a peaceful practice that brings you comfort.

Relaxation audiotapes can provide guidance for the relaxation process. Listening to peaceful, relaxing music is also helpful as you learn to unwind and release the tension. You can make your own tapes of music you find soothing, or you can buy CDs of water sounds, forest sounds, and other mixes you find pleasant.

Guided Imagery and Visualization

This is a form of relaxation exercise in which you focus on a pleasant image. You practice breathing slowly and deeply, and bring up a memory that is peaceful and pleasant.

Focus on the sights, the sounds, the smells—use all your senses to make the image as complete as you can. Once you have an image in your mind, it belongs to you, and you can go to that peaceful place whenever you feel pain.

Guided imagery and visualization are terms that are often used together. Guided simply means that you have help in creating the image that works for you. This help might come from a psychologist or mental health counselor trained in this relaxation technique, but it can also come from an audiotape or CD. If you can conjure up your peaceful place on your own, that works, too!

To practice guided imagery, first find a quiet place without distractions. Get into a comfortable position and take a deep, cleansing breath. Tell yourself that you are safe and relaxed. Next, envision the scene you created and place yourself somewhere in it. If it is a mountain scene, perhaps you are in a snug cabin or fishing on a glacial lake. If it's at the seashore, you are warm and enjoying the tang of the ocean air.

Wherever your place is, it is one of tranquility and safety and, especially, one free from pain. As you learn to call up this place when you need it, you should notice your tension and stress slipping away.

Some people take another tack and picture their pain as something tangible, like a stone, that they can cast away from themselves. Perhaps you can imagine your pain encased in a balloon that you release into the atmosphere. Whatever you feel right with is right for you.

Consultation

Guided imagery and visualization work because the brain responds in the same way to what is real and to what you have created in your mind. You have the power!

Meditation

Meditation is another relaxation technique that can help relieve the pain of arthritis by easing muscle tension. Meditation redirects your awareness or mindfulness away from pain. It allows you to refocus and concentrate your thinking through visualization, relaxation, and proper breathing. Twenty minutes of meditation is considered a good time span to aim for, although you may find it easier to begin with three- or four-minute time blocks with a one-minute break between them.

You may think that meditation belongs to the yoga experts, sitting cross-legged on their mats, palms outstretched, thumb and index finger forming a circle, murmuring "ohmmmm." This is the Hollywood version. Meditation doesn't have to be a spectacle, and it doesn't require an advanced knowledge of yoga. Actually, meditation is like everything else. Once you learn how to do it, it's easy. Children can and do meditate, and meditation can be a helpful practice for children with juvenile arthritis.

In meditation you clear your mind, letting go of all your stress and pain. How you focus your attention is up to you. Whether you use a particular syllable for your *mantra* ("om," for example), visualize a peaceful scene, or concentrate on your breathing, the result is the same: clearing your mind of stressors to achieve a relaxed physical state—a place without pain.

def•i•ni•tion

A **mantra** is something that protects the mind. It's your personal creation. Reciting your mantra removes all outside distractions and encourages you to relax and become at peace.

Choose whatever posture is most relaxing and comfortable for you. You may meditate with your eyes open or closed, but open is the preferred way. Do not focus on any one specific thing. Your mouth should be slightly open. One classic way of practicing meditation is to follow your breath. Exhale deeply a few times to allow the carbon dioxide to clear from your lungs. Then imagine that a lotus flower lives in your lower belly. Inhale slowly and feel the blossom expand. Exhale slowly and feel the blossom gently close.

Another method for practicing meditation is to allow yourself to contemplate a religious icon, a crystal, a flower, or some other object that has a positive connection with you. Just let yourself *be* in calm attention to this object.

Meditation is both a practice and a state of being. Learning how to use meditation to arrive at a meditative state takes time and practice. It can't be rushed. Even the experts, those yogis who have meditated for a lifetime, may only rarely approach a truly meditative state. Regardless, the benefits of meditation still hold and you may find that this practice helps you deal with your arthritis pain.

Spirituality and Prayer

With many relaxation techniques, the goal is to distract the mind from thinking about pain. Spirituality and prayer, however, take pain management to a different plane.

For people who pray, there is a real sense of turning over life's problems to God, the Higher Power. Whether you ask for strength to persevere, relief from pain, or spiritual comfort, prayer can be a powerful addition to medications and physical therapy. It's a reassurance that you are connected to something much bigger than yourself, a Supreme Being who cares for you.

Faith is something that cannot be scientifically dissected or proven. By definition, faith is the belief in things not seen. For someone who prays, it isn't necessary to have concrete proof of how prayer works. It's enough to know that it does.

For those who do not have a particular religious affiliation, spirituality can offer many of the same advantages. Spirituality doesn't require belief in a God or gods; it simply makes the connection of self with something greater. This can be nature, or life, or the greater good.

If you feel your pain controls you, then you are a victim of your pain and have no power to deal with it. Just as with prayer, spirituality involves relinquishing control to a higher power. Letting go of the illusion of control can mean letting go of the pain.

Breathing

Every breath you take can reinforce your pain or can help you channel your energies away from it. The trick is in learning how to breathe for maximum benefit.

Slow, regulated breathing is an essential component of relaxation. In fact, it's impossible to relax if your breathing is shallow and rapid—the kind of breathing that comes with pain and is aggravated by stress, anxiety, and worry.

Learning how to breathe properly can give you more control over your pain. If you're doing it right, you'll notice that your lower abdomen is gently rising and falling in rhythm.

To practice deep breathing, inhale through your nose and exhale through your mouth. As you do this, your muscles will relax, decreasing tension. The oxygen supply to your body's cells increases and this helps produce endorphins, the body's feel-good hormones. Your mind will perceive this relaxed state, and you'll feel less pain.

Consultation

Endorphins are also produced during exercise and help explain what athletes call the "runner's high." Endorphins are opioids, produced by the brain, spinal cord, and other parts of the body. Endorphins act as analgesics—they're natural pain-killers.

A Sense of Humor

Your mind-set can have a great deal to do with how severely you perceive your pain. If you've been blessed with an optimistic outlook on life, you've got a head start, but it's never too late to cultivate a sense of humor. Try to see the absurd, the weird, and the odd moments along your path in life. Arthritis isn't funny, but there are times when you'll find that having a sense of humor can put arthritis in its place.

How does humor work? It takes away the fear of the unknown and strips arthritis of its power to control how you feel. Humor allows you to keep a sense of perspective. But there's more! Research has proven that laughter and humor boost your immune system, improve your circulation, and—of importance to arthritis sufferers—help manage chronic pain.

Norman Cousins, the political journalist, professor, and author, suffered from a type of arthritis known as ankylosing spondylitis (see Chapter 6). Medicine was not relieving his pain, so he set out on his own to see how humor might help. He figured he had nothing to lose. He watched funny movies and read humorous books. What he found surprised him and his doctors as well. Cousins found that ten minutes of laughter resulted in two hours of pain-free sleep. Impressed with the results, he continued his laughter therapy until he could sleep through most of the night.

> **Straight Talk**
>
> My father told me once that the same fire that melts wax makes steel. I didn't understand it then, but now I do. It's all about how we react to what life throws at us that makes all the difference.
>
> —Ben, age 45, diagnosed with ankylosing spondylitis at age 32

Blood tests confirmed that his inflammation had indeed decreased, so not only was Norman Cousins *feeling* better, he was also *getting* better. He was one of the first prominent people to show how the mind-body connection could help relieve pain. Cousins wasn't defeated by his arthritis pain; rather, he was motivated by it. Try it for yourself. You've got nothing to lose and potentially a great deal to gain.

Support Groups

"I know just how you feel." If you've heard this from a family member or well-meaning friend, you know how frustrating it can be. Unless someone is speaking from experience, words meant to be comforting can be aggravating instead.

Support groups, however, are made up of people who really *do* know just how you feel. And no matter what kind of arthritis you have, there is a group that can help you cope. Support groups offer information, resources, and comfort, and they speak with the voice of experience. There are two main kinds of support groups: those that meet on a regular basis at a specific location and those that meet online. Each kind of group has advantages.

If you have transportation or mobility issues, then a virtual group may be just what you're looking for. They're available 24 hours a day. You don't have to wait until the next scheduled meeting if something has come up that you want to discuss—you can be sure that whenever you want to talk to someone, somebody will be online. Another asset of the virtual option is the larger pool of people available to talk with. With greater numbers come more diverse experiences and more potential that you'll find the answer or information you're looking for.

With the more traditional type of group, there's the opportunity to make face-to-face connections. You can develop real friendships, and the smaller size of the group tends to lead to tighter bonds. The regular schedule of meetings may be what you need to get yourself out and about. And being able to help others answer their questions will also give your ego a nice boost.

You don't have to settle for one or the other, however. Perhaps a combination of the two kinds of groups will give you the support you need on a schedule that works for you.

Your rheumatologist may be able to connect you with a support group for your particular form of arthritis. Also, check with your local hospital. The Arthritis Foundation can provide you with a list of support groups in your area (www.arthritis.org).

The Least You Need to Know

- Perceptions of pain are unique to each individual.
- Stress can increase the pain of arthritis.
- You can manage your pain with self-help strategies such as keeping a pain diary.
- Relaxation techniques such as guided imagery and meditation can help relieve arthritis pain.
- Humor, distraction, and proper breathing are your allies.
- Support groups provide knowledge and resources as well as moral support.

Chapter 15

Fighting Fatigue

In This Chapter

- ◆ Why do you feel so tired?
- ◆ Sorting through the potential causes
- ◆ Talking to your rheumatologist
- ◆ Promoting restful sleep
- ◆ Is it a sleep disorder?
- ◆ Cleaning up your act: sleep hygiene

If you are coping with arthritis, you are fighting fatigue. It's a symptom of many types of arthritis and related conditions. This fatigue has many causes, and in this chapter you'll discover what they are and how to combat them and regain your energy.

A Common Symptom

Along with pain and stiffness, fatigue ranks at the top of the list of symptoms for arthritis and other rheumatologic conditions. It is now receiving some serious attention from researchers.

At George Mason University in Fairfax, Virginia, researchers have targeted fatigue as a focus for their studies.

> ### Straight Talk
>
> If you interview people with chronic illnesses, they will tell you that they suffer from fatigue. And by suffer, they mean they notice it interferes with their normal, customary, and desired activities.
>
> —Dr. Lynn Gerber (Director of the Center for the Study of Chronic Illness and Disability at George Mason University)

The December 1999 issue of the journal *MEDSURG Nursing*, the official publication of the Academy of Medical-Surgical Nurses, reported on a study of fatigue in patients with chronic illness. Researchers found that fatigue was an important component of how people perceived their health status.

A person's level of fatigue could be used as a measuring tool to identify individuals who were at high risk for negative changes in their perceptions of how illness affected their lives. Researchers recommended identifying the fatigue level of a patient as a standard part of a comprehensive assessment so that appropriate interventions could be put in place.

Fatigue: The Messenger

When you're feeling washed out, drained, and exhausted, and even getting up out of your chair begins to take on the monumental proportions of climbing Everest, it's time to get to the root of your fatigue and take measures to regain your energy.

You've undoubtedly heard that pain is your body telling you that something is wrong. This is true, of course. Pain is a signal designed to get you to act and do something about the source of the pain.

Fatigue is also a message sent to you courtesy of your body. Fighting inflammation is tough work, and your body expends much energy in the battle. Your body is using so much energy to combat the pain that fatigue is the natural result. Your body needs rest. There's just nothing left in the reserves, and the result is that you feel spent. It's a natural response, but it can be frustrating when you have other work that needs to be done.

Fatigue and Flares

You may notice that during periods of increased disease activity, or flares, your fatigue increases. Fatigue is a result of the body's reaction to substances released in the bloodstream by activated immune cells.

Fatigue is a characteristic of autoimmune diseases, such as the inflammatory types of arthritis—so much so that the absence of fatigue in people with rheumatoid arthritis is considered to be one indicator that the disease is in remission. Conversely, an increase in fatigue can signal the onset of a flare. Fatigue is strongly associated with decreased ability to function and with an increase in symptoms of depression. It's also the most common symptom of systemic lupus erythematosus (SLE) or lupus, as it's commonly called (see Chapter 8).

Pinpointing the Causes of Fatigue

You know that fatigue is a common symptom of chronic illness and you know how fatigue can interrupt your life, but getting to the root of your fatigue can help you treat it and get back some energy.

Just as everyone's symptoms are different and everyone's experience with arthritis is different, so are the causes of fatigue. The cause could be medical, related to your medication, a result of your sleep (or lack of sleep) habits, or something entirely different. It can take some investigative work on your part, and on the part of your rheumatologist, to arrive at the answer.

Are You Anemic?

If you have a form of inflammatory arthritis, such as rheumatoid arthritis (RA), it's quite possible that you are anemic. This means that your red blood cell count is too low. Fatigue is a symptom of anemia, and the severity of your fatigue relates to the severity of your anemia.

Anemia is a symptom of RA, affecting up to two thirds of people with this condition. If this anemia is treated successfully, other symptoms, such as pain, swelling, and tenderness, also respond better to treatment. A decrease in fatigue and an increase in energy are a bonus.

Your blood contains red cells, white cells, and platelets. The white cells fight infection, platelets allow your blood to clot, and red cells contain hemoglobin, a protein that allows them to transport oxygen. Your body's tissues need oxygen to function, and the amount of oxygen they get depends upon how much oxygen your red blood cells are transporting.

What causes anemia? There are a variety of causes, but if you have arthritis you may have some blood loss from your gastrointestinal tract caused by your arthritis medications. Also, bone marrow changes can occur with inflammatory arthritis, and these changes can prevent the release of iron into your red blood cells.

Consultation

Hemoglobin is also a pigment, and it gives these cells their red color. Red blood cells are also called erythrocytes.

To determine if you have anemia, your physician will take a blood sample and send it to a medical laboratory for analysis. The test is called a complete blood count (CBC), and that's exactly what the lab does—it counts the number of blood cells in a sample of your blood and then compares the result with an average range. The red blood cell count is part of that CBC.

Anemia can be treated. If your test results indicate that you do have anemia, your rheumatologist may prescribe medication to treat it, along with iron supplements, if indicated.

Chronic Pain

Arthritis is a chronic disease, and the pain that accompanies arthritis is chronic as well. Pain is an energy zapper. Chapter 14 covered some strategies for managing pain, and in this section, we'll take a look at how pain contributes to fatigue.

First of all, pain causes you to reduce your activity. It hurts to move, and so you don't. The problem with that solution is that lack of movement actually intensifies your symptoms and leads to an increase in fatigue. Getting up and moving, even when it's not on your preferred activity list, can actually increase your energy. This is why a program of regular, mild to moderate exercise is part of your arthritis-fighting prescription and part of your fatigue-fighting prescription, as well.

Second, pain interferes with the quality of sleep. You may have difficulty getting to sleep because you can't get comfortable. When you do drift off, you may awaken because of your pain. It's a common misconception that sleep becomes more elusive as we age, and so you may attribute your broken sleep patterns to the aging process, when in reality, they're directly connected to arthritis. You hurt, you're not sleeping, and if you don't get this problem resolved, you're going to suffer the effects of sleep deprivation.

Pain that wakes you during the night may be the result of your pain medication wearing off. Your rheumatologist may adjust your dosage or prescribe a different medication to correct this problem.

Sleep Deprivation

A 2006 study by researchers at the University of California, Los Angeles, evaluated the effects of sleep deprivation on 30 healthy adults. Researchers found that after only one night, participants who were kept awake from 11 P.M. to 3 A.M. experienced an increase in inflammatory chemicals, the chemicals produced by the body in autoimmune diseases, such as rheumatoid arthritis.

Results of a national survey conducted by researchers at the University of North Carolina at Chapel Hill were reported in the February 2000 issue of *Archives of Family Medicine*. This study surveyed 937 Medicare recipients, aged 65 and older, who were asked how they sought relief from arthritis and how arthritis affected them. About one third of the study's participants cited a correlation between arthritis and sleep loss.

> **Straight Talk**
>
> Just let me get a good night's sleep and I can handle just about anything. You really don't want to be around me if I'm not sleeping well.
>
> —Joe, age 48, diagnosed with lupus

It's a self-perpetuating cycle. Lack of good sleep leads to increased perception of pain, irritability, problems with concentration, and, surprisingly, weight gain. Since weight gain puts extra stress on your joints, it also contributes to pain and inflammation, and the vicious cycle continues.

You know that losing weight, and even maintaining your weight, becomes more difficult with age. You can do everything right, however, and still find the scales creeping up. Why does this happen? It can be a result of sleep deprivation.

A recently published analysis of the Nurses' Health Study found that, among the nearly 70,000 women in the study, those who slept no more than six hours nightly faced a 12 percent higher likelihood of gaining 33 pounds during the 16-year study. The risk was 32 percent higher if they slept five hours or less.

This weight gain had nothing to do with increased calorie consumption, either. These women didn't take in any additional calories above those required to maintain a normal weight. There aren't any definitive answers as to why this happened, but one theory is that sleep deprivation may alter the body's metabolism.

Consultation _____

Two hormones, leptin and grehlin, help your body with appetite control and regulate your weight. When lack of sleep becomes a chronic problem, grehlin (which increases your appetite) levels rise and leptin (which keeps your appetite under control) levels fall. It doesn't seem to matter if you exercise and watch your diet. Sleep deprivation may contribute to weight gain.

The Medication Connection

Some medications used to treat arthritis may have adverse effects on your sleep. They may keep you awake at night or cause you to feel sleepy during the day. For example, celecoxib (Celebrex) has insomnia listed as a possible side effect, and methotrexate, prednisone, and hydroxychloroquine, often prescribed to treat rheumatoid arthritis, may negatively affect your sleep.

What can you do to increase your chances of a good night's rest? Taking these prescriptions in the morning rather than in the evening can help. Both your rheumatologist and your pharmacist are good sources of information about medication interactions and possible adverse side effects. It's essential to understand your medications. Read the labels and ask questions. This is all part of becoming an active member of your healthcare team.

Some pain medications list drowsiness as a possible side effect. These include oxycodone (OxyContin); some prescription nonsteroidal anti-inflammatory drugs (NSAIDs), such as diclofenac (Voltaren) or naproxen (Naprosyn); tricyclic antidepressants such as amitriptyline hydrochloride (Elavil); and disease-modifying antirheumatic drugs (DMARDs) such as azathioprine (Imuran). If you are experiencing drowsiness during the day or difficulty falling asleep at night, check with your rheumatologist or pharmacist. Do not stop your medications without talking to your doctor first. Abruptly stopping medications, especially selective serotonin reuptake inhibitors (SSRIs), or missing several doses can lead to a condition known as "discontinuation syndrome."

Depression and Fatigue

You may not have considered the relationship of depression to your fatigue, but it's definitely worth investigating. Depression is not "all in your head," as you may have heard. Rather, it's a recognized medical condition with specific, characteristic symptoms. Often, depression comes along with other medical conditions, such as arthritis, as an uninvited guest—a guest that overstays his welcome and resists all your efforts to evict him.

Researchers at the University of North Carolina at Chapel Hill were interested in learning how frequently RA patients discussed depression with their rheumatologists. They found that almost 11 percent of people with RA had symptoms of moderate to severe depression, but only 1 in 5 talked to their doctors about it. The level of depression increased in people whose normal activities had been restricted by RA. The study was reported in the February 2008 issue of *Arthritis Care & Research*.

Depression is often associated with chronic illness, as we discussed in Chapter 13. It can develop as part of the disease process itself, as a reaction to certain medications, or in conjunction with lifestyle changes forced upon you by that chronic illness. It's important to recognize the symptoms of depression, because depression can be treated.

Fatigue is a hallmark symptom of depression, and if your fatigue is accompanied by changes in your sleep patterns, appetite changes, and a general feeling of hopelessness, talk to your doctor. Symptoms lasting more than two weeks may be caused by depression.

There are a wide variety of medications available to treat depression, but daytime drowsiness is a possible side effect of certain antidepressant medications. Up to 20 percent of patients taking selective serotonin reuptake inhibitor (SSRI) antidepressants, such as Paxil, Prozac, or Zoloft, report drowsiness as a side effect. This is an issue to discuss with your rheumatologist. Changing your dosage or the time of day you take this medication can solve the problem.

Stress and Fatigue

Coping with chronic illness produces stress. The stress doesn't diminish—it hangs around and can build until you're mentally, emotionally, and physically exhausted. Chapter 13 discusses stress in greater detail. Learning stress management techniques is one way to reduce the fatigue that stress can bring. Regular exercise for your body (but not close to bedtime) coupled with meditation and other relaxation strategies (covered later in this chapter) for your mind can help.

Feeling Good Today—Let's Overdo It!

After you've gone through a flare and come out on the other side, you can feel the need to make up for lost time. You plunge into tasks that have piled up while you weren't able to attend to them. And still it seems to take longer than it should. Arthritis forces you to go more slowly than you'd like. So you push on and try to ignore the pain and stiffness. The next day you can hardly move. What went wrong?

It's easy to mistake a little bit of energy for much more than it is and reality doesn't hit until you're well into an activity that won't let you quit. But there's just one way to cope, and that's to pace yourself.

Not everything needs to be done immediately, and not everything worth doing is worth doing perfectly. Sometimes good enough is good enough. There's always another day, and you'll never run out of work. Understand that, for now, energy is a limited resource. Learn to plan ahead and prioritize and you'll conserve your energy.

Talking to Your Rheumatologist About Fatigue

"I just feel tired all the time." You're likely to report that to your rheumatologist and then sit back and wait for him to do something about it. To be fair, he needs a little more information. Just as arriving at your diagnosis of arthritis or a related rheumatic disorder involved ruling out other possibilities, getting to the root of your fatigue works the same way. Is your fatigue caused by a flare, your medications, or a sleep disorder?

It can take a little time to find a solution that will work for you. And just as with your initial diagnosis, certain tests can point to some possible causes:

- ◆ **White blood cell count (WBC).** If this level is high, it may indicate the presence of an infection. If your body is fighting an infection, it's using extra energy, and this can make you feel tired. It's your body telling you to rest and conserve energy.

- ◆ **Thyroid-stimulating hormone test (TSH).** A TSH level that is too low means that the thyroid gland (which regulates your metabolism) isn't producing enough hormone. This condition is called hypothyroidism, and fatigue is a symptom. Hypothyroidism occurs more often in people with autoimmune disorders, such as rheumatoid arthritis.

- ◆ **Pulse oximetry test.** This is a simple test that measures oxygen levels in the blood. Blood that is not well saturated with oxygen can cause fatigue. Lung disorders or a condition such as sleep apnea can deplete oxygen from your blood.

◆ **Urinalysis.** Urine can be tested to see if bacteria, excess protein, or blood is present. Fatigue may be related to a urinary tract infection, kidney problems, or metabolic disorders, such as anemia or diabetes.

If these tests rule out certain obvious causes, it may be time to consider other possibilities.

Self-Help Strategies

First of all, exercise. Mild to moderate regular exercise can promote more restful sleep. You'll strengthen your muscles around your affected joints and that will help you move with less pain. Less pain = better sleep. Also, there's the endorphin release that comes with exercise. Endorphins are produced by your brain and help relieve pain. For more information on exercise, including the types that are appropriate if you have arthritis, see Chapter 17.

Watch your diet. Food fuels your body, so choose foods that are packed with nutrients and help your body fight the symptoms of arthritis. A Mediterranean-type diet is a good one to follow, and you can find details in Chapter 16.

Use labor-saving devices to avoid wearing yourself out. Your occupational therapist has a catalog full of items that can help you accomplish tasks and conserve energy at the same time. Also, use your braces or splints to support your joints. This will help decrease fatigue.

The Stages of Sleep

It seems simple enough. You're exhausted, so you decide to rest. That's good, but rest isn't sleep. Scientists aren't exactly sure about all the purposes of sleep, but they do know it's a time for renewing the body's energy supply. To get restful, restorative sleep, however, your body needs to move among the different stages of sleep:

◆ **Stage 1.** This is the transition from wakefulness to real sleep.

◆ **Stage 2.** This is light sleep but is considered the first stage of true sleep.

◆ **Stage 3.** This is moderately deep sleep, characterized by deep, slow brain waves.

◆ **Stage 4.** This is the deepest stage of sleep. It's difficult to waken people from this level. It's the restorative stage, and if you have a sleep disorder, this is the level that's of concern. These first four stages are called non-REM sleep.

◆ **REM sleep.** REM stands for *rapid eye movement*, and this is when you dream. After about 10 minutes of REM sleep, your brain begins the sleep cycle over again. Each cycle lasts about 90 minutes.

def•i•ni•tion

Insomnia refers both to a difficulty in falling asleep as well as difficulty in staying asleep. The word literally means "without sleep."

If pain, medications, stress, or any other agent interferes with your sleep cycle, you're going to be fatigued, no matter how many hours you spend in bed. It's important to make the most of your mattress time and deal with *insomnia*.

Most people need between seven and nine hours of sleep a night, so if nighttime has become awake time, it's important to discuss your sleep problems with your physician.

Sleep Disorders and Daytime Fatigue

There's a big difference between feeling sleepy and feeling tired. If you can fall asleep easily or if you find yourself dozing off unintentionally during the day, you may have a condition known as excessive daytime sleepiness (EDS), also referred to as hypersomnia.

If sleep is the farthest thing from your mind, but you feel physically tired, you have fatigue and you may or may not have a sleep disorder. If you have rheumatoid arthritis, ankylosing spondylitis, Sjögren's syndrome, or lupus, you understand how overwhelming fatigue can be.

Restless Legs Syndrome

Restless legs syndrome (RLS) is the unrelenting urge to move your legs to relieve an overwhelming unpleasant sensation. Once you move your legs, the sensation stops for a time, but shortly afterward, that unpleasant sensation returns. It's maddening and keeps you awake as the hours tick by. RLS is common in Sjögren's syndrome.

Another sleep spoiler is periodic limb movement disorder (PLMD). This condition causes cramps and movements of your limbs while you're asleep. You may not know that you're constantly moving your arms and legs until your bed partner tells you. It's common to have PLMD if you have RLS, but most PLMD sufferers don't have RLS.

Sometimes the cause of these problems is iron deficiency, and taking prescribed iron supplements can ease the symptoms. Other causes include caffeine, selective serotonin reuptake inhibitors (SSRIs) and tricyclic antidepressants, and uremia.

Sleep Apnea

This condition literally means *without breath*. There are three types of apnea: obstructive, central, and mixed, with obstructive being the most common. While the three types have different root causes, each can be characterized by stopped breathing. People with sleep apnea regularly stop breathing while they sleep, sometimes hundreds of times during the night and often for a minute or longer at a time.

The American Sleep Apnea Association (www.sleepapnea.org) explains that obstructive sleep apnea (OSA) is caused by a blockage of the airway, usually when the soft tissue in the rear of the throat collapses and closes during sleep. In central sleep apnea, the airway is not blocked, but the brain fails to signal the muscles to breathe. Mixed apnea is a combination of the two. With each apnea event, your brain briefly arouses you so you can resume breathing, but consequently your sleep is extremely fragmented and of poor quality.

Sleep apnea affects more than 12 million Americans, according to the National Institutes of Health, and is present in 12 percent of individuals with ankylosing spondylitis. Untreated sleep apnea can be life-threatening.

Sleep apnea can be treated with a *CPAP* machine that blows a fixed amount of air through your airways during the night, keeping them open so you don't snort and gasp, but instead get a good night's sleep.

Just as there are pain clinics to help you manage your pain, sleep clinics can help you manage your sleep problems. The first step in reclaiming a good night's sleep is to take a serious look at your sleep habits.

def•i•ni•tion

CPAP stands for *continuous positive airway pressure.* The CPAP device is worn on your face and secured with straps around your head.

Keeping a Sleep Diary

Your physician will most likely ask you to keep a sleep diary for a couple of weeks to help pinpoint the issues that are causing your sleep difficulties. To get the most benefit from it, you'll need to be honest and accurate and faithfully record everything it asks for.

You can download sample sleep diaries off the Internet, but all you really need is a small spiral notebook, a pen, and a clock by your bedside. If you're having trouble sleeping, you probably check the clock on your nightstand frequently, but now there will be a purpose to it! Here's what a sample day might look like:

Monday: Woke up at 4:00 A.M. Couldn't get back to sleep. Got out of bed at 6:00.

6:00   *drank cup of coffee*

7:00   *took medication [enter the name and dosage]*

8:30   *drank cup of coffee*

9:00   *exercised 30 minutes on treadmill*

12:00 P.M.   *drank caffeinated beverage*

4:00   *took medication [enter the name and dosage]*

5:30   *drank martini (1½ oz. gin)*

10:00   *went to bed, but couldn't fall asleep*

12:00 A.M.   *still awake*

1:30 (approximate)   *fell asleep*

You'll keep a record like this for two weeks, entering times and amounts of caffeine, alcohol, and exercise. You'll undoubtedly need to estimate when you finally do fall asleep.

Sleep Hygiene

At your next doctor appointment, bring that diary along and discuss the information with your physician. He'll then be able to give you specific suggestions you can implement and may give you some information on sleep hygiene, specific practices you can employ to help you get a better night's sleep. What's sleep hygiene all about? Basically, it's about cleaning up your pre-bedtime routines.

◆ Establish a regular sleep/wake schedule and keep to it as much as possible. By training your body to anticipate sleep, you'll be priming the pump, and you will begin to feel sleepy as your bedtime approaches. If you haven't fallen asleep after 20 minutes, get up and read or do something else relaxing until you feel tired.

◆ Limit your intake of alcohol. A nightcap may help you fall asleep but will interfere with your ability to stay asleep.

◆ Stick to decaffeinated beverages as nighttime approaches. Caffeine is a stimulant, and a stimulant will keep you awake.

◆ Make your bedroom a place that invites sleep. That means no television or computer. Don't do work in bed. Reserve your bed exclusively for sleep and sex (which can help you sleep!).

Precautions

If your body is sensitive to the effects of caffeine, add chocolate to your list of foods and drinks to avoid at night. Chocolate contains caffeine!

◆ Keep your sleeping quarters darkened and cool. Light can interfere with your sleep, telling your brain that it's time to wake up.

◆ A light snack before retiring can prevent hunger from waking you during the night.

◆ Start to reframe your thinking about bedtime. Adopt a positive attitude, instead of reinforcing the thought that this is just one more night you're not going to be able to sleep. Keep conversations light and avoid stress for two to three hours before retiring.

◆ Take a warm bath or listen to relaxing music before going to bed.

◆ Spend some quiet time alone and read for pleasure before bedtime.

Give yourself some time to adapt to your new pre-bedtime habits and you'll likely see some improvement in your ability to fall asleep and stay asleep.

In older adults, practicing sleep hygiene might not be enough to change sleep patterns. This is where a sleep specialist can help. A sleep specialist can teach you specific strategies that can break ingrained habits that are keeping you from falling and staying asleep. The following tips are from the Arthritis Foundation:

◆ **Stimulus control.** Similar to the sleep hygiene tip, you only enter your bedroom to sleep or for sex. If you can't sleep, you leave and go into another room until you're tired. Regardless of how little you've slept, you rise at the same time every day.

◆ **Sleep restriction.** If you fall asleep easily but can't stay asleep, this may help. To begin, you reduce the amount of time you spend asleep by going to bed 15 minutes later than usual. If your sleep doesn't improve after a week, add another 15 minutes. Don't go to bed earlier, even if you're tired. In the short term you're experiencing more sleep depriviation, but you're retraining your body. When you start seeing some improvement, go to be 15 minutes earlier. The short-term result is more sleep deprivation, but the goal is to help sleep correct itself, with wakeful periods decreasing. As your sleep improves, start going to bed 15 minutes earlier. The Arthritis Foundation advises that you shouldn't go below 5 hours of sleeping—or trying to sleep!

◆ **Relaxation techniques.** Alternately tensing and relaxing muscles can help relieve anxiety.

◆ **Paradoxical intention.** If your problem is falling asleep, this is a psychological approach. You reduce your anxiety about your lack of sleep by telling yourself you're going to stay awake instead of going to sleep. It becomes harder and harder to stay awake, so you fall asleep.

◆ **Cognitive restructuring.** Instead of worrying that you're not going to fall asleep and envisioning tomorrow as another day filled with fatigue, you picture yourself rested and unstressed because you've well rested.

As an adjunct to all of these strategies, if it becomes necessary, your doctor can prescribe a sleeping medication to help you establish a better sleeping pattern. These aren't permanent solutions, however, they're just to help you get started on the road to restful sleep. These newer medications, including eszopiclone (Lunesta), lorazepam (Ativan), zaleplon (Sonata), and zolpidem (Ambien), may be less likely to trigger low-dose dependence than older sleep medications or mild tranquilizers, such as alprazolam (Xanax), clonazepam (Klonopin), and diazepam (Valium).

Even if a medication isn't physically addictive, it can be psychologically addictive. To help avoid this, take sleeping medications only when prescribed and only for as long as your physician recommends.

Precautions

If you smoke, stop. A recent study found that even healthy cigarette smokers are four times more likely than nonsmokers to report feeling as though they did not get a restful night's sleep.

If you are considering an over-the-counter sleeping medication, check with your physician first. They may contain antihistamines or acetaminophen. In the first case, you may feel wiped out the next day. In the latter case, you may be exceeding your recommended dosage if your rheumatologist has already prescribed it for you. That could lead to liver problems.

Two popular supplements used to promote sleep are melatonin and valerian. Melatonin is a hormone made by the body that helps regulate its internal clock, and melatonin supplements are a synthetic form of that hormone. Valerian is an herb. Neither of these supplements is recommended for long-term use, and more research needs to be done to determine both their safety and their efficacy.

Fatigue is a complex symptom with many contributing factors. Stress, insomnia, increased disease activity, and overexertion can all play a part, but fighting fatigue will help you manage your arthritis more successfully.

The Least You Need to Know

- ◆ Stress, flares, anemia, depression, and many other factors can contribute to a feeling of fatigue.

- ◆ Your rheumatologist can work with you to determine the cause of your fatigue.

- ◆ Planning ahead and prioritizing tasks can help you conserve energy, which is your first step toward fighting fatigue.

- ◆ Flares, pain, and stress can work together to rob you of restful sleep. Talk to your rheumatologist about ways to manage this.

- ◆ Practicing sleep hygiene can help you get restorative sleep and reduce daytime fatigue.

Chapter 16

Nutrition and Weight Management

In This Chapter

- ◆ Going easy on your joints
- ◆ Simple nutrition
- ◆ Avoiding foolish fads
- ◆ Putting it all together
- ◆ Streamlining your kitchen to make cooking easier

When you are hurting, it can take a Herculean effort to prepare nutritious meals. But if you turn to the fast-food fix, the results are added pounds that put strain on inflamed joints and a host of other unwelcome problems. In this chapter, you'll learn some simple tricks for eating well and keeping your weight under control, along with tips on streamlining food preparation, shopping, and your kitchen.

Your Weight and Arthritis

Maintaining a proper weight is essential for relieving stress on inflamed joints. Carrying around additional weight slows you down, decreases your energy, and increases your risk of diabetes, heart disease, and other medical conditions. Choose your foods wisely and eat in moderation, and your joints (along with the rest of your body) will thank you.

Weight management is simple math. If you take in more calories than you need, you'll gain weight. Take in fewer than you need and you'll lose weight. Strike a happy balance between caloric intake and calories used and you'll maintain your weight.

Precautions

If you are taking corticosteroids to treat your arthritis symptoms, you may experience weight gain. Although steroids can increase your appetite, weight gain is not necessarily the result of extra caloric intake on your part and can be a frustrating side effect of these medications. Fortunately, weight gain isn't that common with the very low doses of corticosteroids usually used to treat rheumatoid arthritis.

Arthritis can make movement painful, causing you to be more sedentary than you otherwise would be. Getting up and moving, however, in the form of mild to moderate regular exercise, can give you more energy and make movement less painful. You'll read more about therapeutic exercise in the next chapter, as breaking out of a sedentary lifestyle is key to managing arthritis pain.

Consuming empty calories is another factor in the weight gain equation. Empty calories fill you up and fill you out, but they don't nourish your body. Examples include soft drinks, candy, and snack foods high in sugar, trans fats, and carbohydrates.

Why do you eat? Understanding your eating patterns is the first step toward managing your weight. Do you eat just because the clock says it's mealtime? Do you eat because you're bored, tired, angry, stressed, or sad? None of these are the right reasons, although many of us give in to them from time to time. It's when these reasons for eating become habit that they can cause us harm.

Keeping a Food Diary

A food diary can be a real eye opener if you're having difficulty controlling your weight. For one week, write down everything you eat. Everything. Don't leave anything out. That spoonful of chocolate ice cream? Count it. That one last cookie in the package? Count it. Also write down the time of day that you ate and how you were feeling at the time.

You may be surprised to see that those odds and ends and tidbits add up to some serious calories over the course of the week. And maybe you didn't even really taste them or enjoy them. You just ate them because they were there. The food diary will help you understand your eating patterns, along with the emotional reasons why you're eating.

If you find that you're a fast food addict, you're not alone. Fast food is tempting when you're hurting. It's convenient and relatively inexpensive. Breaking the fast food habit can be a challenge, but the rewards for your health and for managing your arthritis make it well worth the initial struggle.

Even if you're not overly enthused about fruits and vegetables, it's time to re-educate your palate and get reacquainted with nature's bounty.

So, what's next? Once you've taken a look at what you eat and when you eat it, you're ready to take some action. Get rid of the junk food. Promise yourself you'll develop some healthier eating habits, and then follow through. Good nutrition doesn't have to be boring, as you'll see shortly.

Consultation

It takes about three weeks to establish a new habit. So don't give up after the first three days and decide you're never going to like apples. Try peaches or pears or plums! Keep at it and you'll emerge victorious.

You don't have to spend a fortune to learn how to eat well. Your local hospital will probably have classes taught by a dietician. You've got a great opportunity to learn good nutrition habits, get positive reinforcement for your commitment to better nutrition, and collect some simple recipes that are doable even with arthritis. The secret to eating well is planning ahead.

How Pain Affects Appetite

Sometimes undereating, not overeating, is the problem. Joint pain, inflammation, and stiffness can make preparing food difficult, so you may not eat as well as you once did. When you experience a flare you may not have much of an appetite, and you may skip meals or just pick at your food.

Certain arthritis medications can affect your appetite, so check with your doctor if you find you are eating less. Sometimes changing the time of day you take your medication can solve the problem, or a change in medication may be in order.

Dealing with a chronic illness can also increase your risk of developing depression. If your appetite has decreased to the point that food doesn't seem worth the trouble of preparing and eating, talk to your doctor. Depression can be treated and you can get your appetite back.

The Arthritis Diet?

According to the Johns Hopkins Arthritis Center, arthritis patients are estimated to spend more than $1 billion each year on unproven treatments for arthritis, including diets. Researchers have looked for a relationship between diet and arthritis since the 1930s, investigating special diets, supplements, and specific foods that are claimed to cure arthritis or relieve its symptoms. So far, most claims remain unproven.

But people keep looking and hoping for a miracle diet. Just as with alternative therapies for arthritis, the placebo effect further confuses the situation. You believe that something will make you better, and so you begin to feel better. Couple that with the nature of arthritis—sudden flares followed by periods of relief, and you can see why diet claims are hard to prove. If you happen to have eaten a "miracle food" just as you were going into a less active phase of your symptoms, the miracle food may get the credit.

Precautions

Beware of individuals with little or no medical training who make unsubstantiated claims about the benefits of certain foods, supplements, or diets. You run the risk of serious and potentially dangerous health consequences if you follow untested advice.

Few controlled research studies and clinical trials have studied the relationship between specific foods and arthritis. What we have learned about diet and arthritis so far generally centers on rheumatoid arthritis. The Mayo Clinic reports that while there's no definitive evidence that certain foods can affect inflammation and joint pain, some studies suggest that oranges and omega-3 fatty acids may offer some relief of rheumatoid arthritis symptoms. More studies are needed to see if this indeed is true. In the meantime, oranges and omega-3 fatty acids are part of a healthy diet, so you can give them a try.

Power of the Pyramid

While there is no specific arthritis diet, one of the simplest ways to improve your nutrition and manage your weight is to increase your intake of fruits, vegetables, and whole grains and reduce your intake of protein, full-fat dairy products, fats, sweets, and convenience foods. The food pyramid makes choosing the right foods easier.

The food pyramid has replaced the old charts showing recommended numbers of servings of various kinds of foods. You can find a variety of slightly different pyramids from different sources. A good place to begin is with MyPyramid (formerly known as the Food Guide Pyramid), developed by the United States Department of Agriculture (USDA) and the Department of Health and Human Services.

Unlike other food pyramids, which are made of stacked blocks, this one is sliced vertically. Each section contains a specific group of foods. Go to www.mypyramid.gov to see the different parts of the pyramid, create menus, track your weight management, and find many other resources for healthy eating. In addition, the USDA provides pyramids centered around different ethnic eating patterns. General guidelines from the government website include ...

- Look for whole grains.
- Eat more dark green and orange vegetables and more dry beans and peas.
- Eat a variety of fruits daily—five or more.
- Choose low-fat or fat-free dairy.
- Choose low-fat or lean meats and poultry.

Another pyramid comes from researchers at the Mayo Clinic. The Mayo Clinic Healthy Weight Pyramid is sliced into horizontal segments, though the principles behind both pyramids are essentially the same. Go to www.mayoclinic.com for more information.

The Mediterranean Diet

The Mediterranean diet isn't something you can buy. It's a way of eating that's typical of people who live in around the Mediterranean Sea. And many of these people live very long, healthy lives. Staples of this diet include ...

- Lots of fruits and vegetables.
- Fish.

- Healthy fats, such as olive oil and canola oil.

- Nuts.

- Red wine.

- Limited amounts of red meat.

Researchers have investigated the health benefits of the Mediterranean diet for people with arthritis. A study conducted by researchers in Glasgow divided 130 women, ranging in age from 30 to 70, and who had had RA an average of eight years, into two groups. The first group was put on a six-week program of weekly two-hour sessions. These sessions included cooking classes and written dietary information. The control group was given written dietary information only.

The results showed that the women with rheumatoid arthritis who kept to a Mediterranean diet for nine months experienced significant pain relief. The study results also found reduced disease activity and cardiovascular risk. This was important, since people with RA are at increased risk of cardiovascular disease.

The researchers concluded that a Mediterranean diet would be a useful addition to a treatment plan using disease-modifying antirheumatic medications (DMARDs) and that it would be easy to implement and popular with patients. The study appeared in the September 2007 issue of the Annals of the Rheumatic Diseases.

Debunking the Diets

If there's a food, you can be pretty sure someone has invented a diet that either uses it or claims it's pure poison. Fad diets don't preach moderation, but instead go to the extremes. The difficulty with a fad diet is that even if it's not going to hurt you, you probably won't be able to sustain it for very long. In the case of harmful fad diets, that's a good thing.

Here's a look at what's currently making the rounds:

- **The No Tomato (or Potatoes or Peppers or Eggplant) Diet.** These plants belong to the nightshade family, and while parts of these plants are poisonous (potato and tomato leaves, for example), the parts that we eat have nutritional value. There's no scientific evidence to support this diet.

- **The Don't Eat Acid Foods Diet.** This diet that frowns on coffee, red meat, sugar, grains, nuts, and citrus is supposed to be followed for one month only. It's deficient in vitamin C, and that's not good. Again, there's no scientific evidence to support this diet.

- ◆ **The Vegetarian Diet.** A gluten-free vegetarian diet, in combination with prescribed medications, may be of some benefit for people with rheumatoid arthritis.

- ◆ **The Increase Your Omega-3 Fatty Acids Diet.** There are health benefits associated with omega-3s; they can lower your bad cholesterol (LDL) and raise your good cholesterol (HDL). Studies have found them, in combination with prescribed medications, to be of benefit for rheumatoid arthritis.

Straight Talk _____

I swear by gin-soaked raisins. I eat a dozen every day.

—Marla, age 54, diagnosed with rheumatoid arthritis

The Straight Talk response? Alcohol can certainly dull your pain, but it's not a wise choice for treating arthritis. Keep the raisins and eliminate the alcohol.

Including Enough Calcium

Calcium is important, particularly because certain medications used for treating arthritis can leach calcium from your bones. The Arthritis Foundation recommends calcium—1,000 mg per day if you're younger than 50 and 1,200 mg if you're older—to keep bones strong and ward off osteoporosis.

Calcium is available in a wide number of foods. Green leafy vegetables; low-fat milk, yogurt, and cheese; and calcium-fortified juice, bread, and cereal are all sources of calcium. Calcium is also available in supplement form.

Read the labels of calcium supplements to be sure you're getting what your body needs. The Arthritis Foundation recommends that you check the amount of elemental calcium in your supplement. That's what your body will actually absorb. Since your body can only absorb 500 mg of calcium at a time, take your supplements in several small doses throughout the day.

Consultation _____

Your body needs vitamin D to use calcium most efficiently, so look for a supplement that contains both vitamins C and D.

Calcium also plays a role in weight management. If you're having difficulty losing weight, look at the amount of calcium in your diet. Studies have found that people who are calcium-deficient are more likely to be overweight. This may be due to the effect of calcium on certain hormones in your body.

In the September/October 2004 issue of *Arthritis Today*, Dr. Robert Heaney, a calcium expert at Creighton University in Omaha, Nebraska, explains that "When the amount of calcium in the diet falls short, the body responds by increasing its level of a hormone that pulls calcium from bone. That hormone also causes fat cells to switch from breaking down fat to storing it. In effect, it appears that a person who doesn't take in enough calcium winds up with hungry fat cells. The evidence linking calcium to body weight is modest but growing."

Fasting

Fasting can be a high-risk activity and there is no research to support it as a treatment for arthritis. Even in patients who did report some pain relief, symptoms returned within one week of returning to a normal diet.

Coffee

Many studies have tried to prove that coffee is harmful to your health, but they keep coming up short. Now it appears that coffee may help in the treatment of gout. Two recent studies seem to indicate, in fact, that the more coffee you drink, the less likely you are to develop gout.

In the first study, researchers at the Arthritis Research Centre of Canada, the University of British Columbia, Brigham and Women's Hospital, Harvard Medical School, and the Harvard School of Public Health conducted a study of 45,869 men older than 40 who had no history of gout at the beginning of the study. They followed up on these study participants over the course of 12 years.

The second study, based on the Third National Health and Nutrition Examination Survey in the United States, was conducted between 1988 and 1994. It included more than 14,000 men and women at least 20 years old.

In the larger study, researchers found that the risk of gout was 40 percent lower than that of men who never drank coffee for men who drank four to five cups of coffee a day. It was 59 percent lower for men who drank six or more cups a day. There was also a modest risk reduction with those who drank decaffeinated coffee. These findings were independent of all other risk factors for gout, including body mass index, history of hypertension, alcohol use, and a diet high in red meat and high-fat dairy foods. Tea drinking and total caffeine intake were both shown to have no effect on the incidence of gout among the participants. The study's findings were featured in the June 2007 issue of *Arthritis & Rheumatism*.

Results of the second study published in the June 2007 issue of *Arthritis Care & Research* showed that levels of uric acid in the blood significantly decreased with increasing coffee intake, but not with increasing tea intake. In addition, there was no association between total caffeine intake from beverages and uric acid levels. If you are a coffee lover, take heart! However, keep in mind that too much of anything, even regular coffee, can have health consequences. Like most things in life, moderation is the key to success.

Alcohol

While moderate consumption of red wine is a pillar of the Mediterranean diet, it's important to understand that alcohol can affect how well arthritis drugs work. As well, it can weaken your bones. And it also adds pounds by putting extra sugar in your diet.

If you drink alcohol and are also taking nonsteroidal anti-inflammatory drugs (NSAIDs), you run the risk of developing stomach and liver problems. If you suffer from gout, alcohol may increase uric acid levels in your blood and work against your medications.

Be honest with your rheumatologist about your alcohol use to get the most out of your arthritis treatment regimen.

Tobacco

If you smoke, you are already aware of all the negative consequences of the habit. Unfortunately, quitting smoking is not easy and not everyone is successful quitting the first time. You can persevere, and there are numerous products on the market to help you quit successfully. Talk to your doctor when you've made the decision to quit smoking. There are medications available to help you through the transition to a smoke-free life.

Precautions _____

The message is clear: if you smoke, and if you test positive for rheumatoid factor, it's in your best interests to quit. That's just one more reason not to smoke!

The evidence linking smoking with rheumatoid arthritis continues to mount, and the link appears to be strongest in men who test positive for rheumatoid factor. Research presented at the 2006 Annual Meeting of the American College of Rheumatology took a look at 16 studies conducted between 1966 and 2005. The researchers found that when the studies were limited to patients who were positive for rheumatoid factor, men who smoked had twice the chance of developing RA than women who did.

Turning Knowledge into Practice

We've covered the basics of nutrition; looked at the kinds of diets making the anti-arthritis rounds; and checked out the relationship of coffee, alcohol, and smoking to arthritis. Putting everything together comes next.

You know you need to eat well, especially when you have arthritis, but the process of food shopping and food preparation can seem like too much work. Fortunately, there are shortcuts to the process and ways to streamline your kitchen.

Food Shopping

One old-time method of food shopping is new again. If you live in a metropolitan area, you may be able to use the delivery services of your favorite supermarket or buy-in-bulk warehouse. You place your order online and they deliver. If you live outside the warehouse's delivery area, numerous other companies provide delivery service.

One familiar example is Schwan's, which has been delivering food for more than 50 years. You can shop online or by phone and have your food delivered to your door. If you spend a little time online, you'll most likely find the right food delivery service to suit your needs.

Consultation _____

If you shop at the same store frequently, make your grocery list fit the traffic pattern of your store. That way you won't have to use extra energy backtracking.

When you do head to the grocery store, go prepared with a list, so you're not tempted to make impulse purchases. (You know not to shop when you're hungry, right?) If you need a motorized shopping cart, use one! Often, a store can provide someone to help you fill your cart, reaching for items above your head or stooping for items at floor level.

Buying presliced fruits and vegetables can save your hands considerable stress and save you time.

Kitchen Makeover

You don't have to do a massive makeover to get the best use of your kitchen. Small changes made a few at a time can reap big dividends and be cost-effective. Bending, lifting, stretching, reaching, stooping, and twisting are motions that will aggravate your arthritis. Finding ways to reduce these motions will make food preparation easier on your joints.

According to the Arthritis Foundation, the triangle can be your best friend in redesigning your kitchen. Your sink, stove (with controls in the front rather than on the back), and refrigerator are the three essential appliances in your kitchen, and they're most efficient when they're about equal distances from one another. If you can work with the triangle shape, keep each side under 8 feet in length for maximum efficiency. (Once you're set with the three essential appliances, you'll undoubtedly want to add a microwave and a dishwasher!) Store kitchen items near the appliance they'll be used with.

In the ideal kitchen, everything would be easily accessible at a counter level that was the ideal for you. But even if that's not realistic, there are modifications you can make that will make cooking easier and more enjoyable:

- ◆ Replace faucets with lifters.
- ◆ Invest in pots and pans with two handles. Cookie sheets come this way as well.
- ◆ Get an automatic jar opener.
- ◆ Install a lazy Susan or pullout shelves in your cabinets.
- ◆ Use tip-out bins for flour and sugar.
- ◆ Store your pots and pans between vertical dividers instead of nesting them.
- ◆ Use lightweight ergonomic cooking utensils.
- ◆ Place nonskid shelf liner underneath mixing bowls to keep them from sliding around the counter.
- ◆ Keep an oven-rack puller on a hook by the stove and use it to save your hands.

Keep items you use frequently within easy reach. Store heavier items lower and lighter items higher. A reach extender is a rod with a trigger-controlled grasp at the far end that will extend your reach by 26 to 30 inches. One can help you fish something from the back of a cupboard or from a shelf above your head.

Now You're Cooking

Make optimum use of your microwave, food processor, and slow cooker. Cook once on days when you're feeling well and make extra meals you can freeze for later. Just be sure not to overdo it and end up exhausted. Take breaks while you're working. And while you're preparing food, why not sit down? Get an adjustable-height ergonomic office chair and cook in comfort. Use a rolling pizza slicer or a rocker knife to do the chopping and save stress on your hands.

Vegetables and cheeses come already shredded, sliced, and diced in handy zip-seal packages. Watch the packaging, however. Some packages with vacuum seals require dynamite to get them open. You want the ones with the press-closure strip.

When you're boiling potatoes or other foods, put them inside a colander basket or deep-fry basket in the pot. You'll be able to lift them out when they're done without having to wrestle with a pot full of boiling water. Add water to the pot via a hose hooked up to your sink's spray nozzle.

Consultation

Use two arms and two hands when you're lifting or carrying. This takes excess strain off painful joints in your elbows, shoulders, hands, and wrists.

And be sure to look for the Arthritis Foundation Ease-of-Use Commendation Logo the next time you are in the grocery store. This seal signifies user-friendly products and packaging.

Remember, if you need it, someone has probably made it. Search online and you'll most likely find the helpful product you're looking for. Also check with your physical therapist and occupational therapist for more ideas. They have catalogues of adaptive devices that can make cooking much easier on your joints.

The Least You Need to Know

- ◆ Maintaining a healthy weight takes stress off your joints.

- ◆ The Mediterranean diet is a good choice for optimum nutrition.

- ◆ Check out the healthful food tips at www.mypyramid.gov for good eating ideas.

- ◆ Coffee is in and smoking is out!

- ◆ Streamlining your kitchen will conserve your energy and make cooking easier and more enjoyable.

Chapter 17

Therapeutic Exercise and Rest: Partners in Health

In This Chapter

- ◆ Getting moving and feeling better
- ◆ Setting goals and moving ahead
- ◆ Listening to your body
- ◆ Recreational activities count, too!

Previously, doctors believed that exercise was not helpful for treating arthritis and even advised against it, fearing it would harm inflamed joints. Today, however, research has shown that moderate, regular exercise has important benefits for arthritis sufferers. Your joints are meant to move. Finding the right exercise program for you, getting moving, and then keeping moving will help you manage your arthritis.

Benefits of Exercise

It's difficult to come up with just a short list of benefits for exercise. For starters, exercise can reduce pain and stiffness, while increasing flexibility and endurance. As you continue exercising, you'll strengthen the muscles that surround your joints. You may become tired at first, but keeping with your exercise program will increase your energy over the long term. You'll bolster your immune system, as well.

Being overweight can aggravate the symptoms of arthritis, but regular exercise can help you lose those extra pounds and successfully manage your weight afterward.

Finally, regular exercise can raise your spirits and increase your self-esteem. You'll be actively involved in leading a healthier life, and you'll reduce your risk of experiencing the symptoms of depression.

Beginning an Exercise Program

There's definitely more involved in a successful exercise program than lacing up your walking shoes and heading out the door. You've got to be psychologically ready and primed to begin if you're going to be successful.

Consultation

According to the Johns Hopkins Arthritis Center, the goals of an exercise program for people with arthritis need to be directed toward the entire body and not just the joints affected with arthritis. It's a total body experience.

First you'll consult with your physician, who may recommend a physical therapist (PT) to work with you to design a program that will benefit you and your particular type of arthritis. Different types of arthritis benefit from different exercise regimens. It's important to start slowly and build over time.

Your exercise program will generally have three components: flexibility, strength building, and endurance. Each of these components targets a specific joint issue.

Are You Ready?

If exercising is new for you, it's going to take some time before this behavior becomes part of your daily routine. In fact, studies of how people go about adopting new behaviors show that up to 40 percent of people are in what's called a "precontemplative stage." This means they're essentially unaware of the problem (in this case, the need to exercise to improve their arthritis symptoms) and haven't actually thought a whole lot about why change may be necessary. Don't get stuck at the precontemplative stage. If you're in this group, it's going to take a little mental processing before you're convinced change is necessary. Your PT can help you with this.

To get the most benefit from your exercise regimen, you need to start right and learn how to move properly. At your first physical therapy session, the PT will interview you to learn about your particular type of arthritis and specific joint issues.

Next, he'll check your range of motion to see how flexible your joint is. This means finding out just how far you're able to move without pain or stiffness. This requires a demonstration from you and some measurements and mathematical computations on his part.

For example, if you have arthritis in your elbow, you'll demonstrate how far you can move that joint without pain or stiffness. You may do this from a sitting position or while standing. The PT will measure this distance and compare it to a normal value. If your elbow is functioning normally, the action of bringing your lower arm up to your biceps (flexing), covers 150 degrees. Straightening your arm covers 180 degrees. It's all about mathematics!

Consultation

Each joint is capable of certain movements, and when everything is working smoothly, you don't give those movements much thought. For example, you can flex, extend, and rotate your wrists and ankles. You can shrug and rotate your shoulder and use it to raise your arm. Knees, elbows, and hips flex, extend, and rotate, and can move both away from and toward the midline of your body.

Once you've gotten your baseline (what you're capable of doing right now) established, you'll be able to set some realistic goals. Do you want to gain more flexibility? Do you want to strengthen your muscles so you can use your joints for work and leisure activities? Your goals will motivate you to keep at your exercise program. Then, after gathering all this information, your PT will design a program specific to your type of arthritis and your individual needs.

Perhaps you've had joint replacement surgery and need to learn how to use that new joint. You'll need instructions on how to safeguard against injury while you're recovering from surgery. Protecting your joints while you are exercising is important, and your PT will show you how to do this.

Flexibility Exercises

Flexibility exercises are also called stretching or range of motion exercises. These are the foundation of your exercise program, and they'll be the first exercises you do each day. They'll build your confidence and help you warm up safely.

Flexibility exercises get the body moving and the blood flowing to the affected joints. They strengthen the muscles, ligaments, and tendons that support your joints. They also help prevent joint deformities. If your fingers are so stiff in the morning that buttoning your shirt, taking the cap off the toothpaste, or even picking up some change from the counter is almost impossible, you'll benefit from flexibility exercises.

Your physical therapist has three different types of flexibility or range of motion exercises to choose from:

♦ Active exercise is used when you're able to use your joint without assistance. In this type of exercise, you do the work.

♦ Active-assistive exercise is used when you can move your joint but need some help doing so or if you feel pain when you do move your joint. You'll move your joint yourself, but the physical therapist will help you by applying pressure to stabilize the joint.

♦ Passive exercise is used when you can't move your joint on your own. In this case the therapist does the moving for you.

Your therapist will be as gentle as possible, although some discomfort may be unavoidable. In order to increase your range of motion, the joint must be moved beyond the point where you feel discomfort. This movement should not cause residual pain, however. Residual pain is pain that continues after the movement has stopped.

You should try to put each joint through its full range of motion every day. Even though you may be climbing stairs, lifting bags of groceries, or bending to tie your shoes, this isn't enough. Everyday activities don't provide a full range of motion workout.

Precautions _____

When you are experiencing a flare, your regular exercise program may not be the best choice for you. Check with your doctor or PT to find out what kinds of activities won't harm your joints.

Your joints are probably stiffest in the morning, so begin your day with flexibility exercises. These will help release that stiffness and protect your joints by reducing the risk of injury that can come with stiff movements. You'll begin to feel a sense of control over your body, and that will relieve tension, which also contributes to stiffness.

You'll want to work up to about 15 minutes each day with these kinds of exercises. Once you have reached this goal, it's time to consider adding strength-building and endurance exercises to your schedule.

Developing a routine that targets each body area will help you increase your flexibility overall.

If you are new to exercise, if you are getting used to a new joint, or if you've been away from exercise for a while, remember to start slowly and build gradually. Here are some useful tips to help you get the most out of your workout routine:

- Aim for fluid motions; avoid jerky movements.

- Plan your routine to flow from one activity to the next. Group your exercises by positions to conserve your energy.

- Begin with no more than 5 repetitions (reps) of each exercise. Increase this number gradually over a couple of weeks, and aim for 10 reps.

- Do the same number of reps and exercises on each side of your body.

Flexibility exercises don't require any kind of special equipment and they can be done almost anywhere you can find a flat surface roomy enough to permit you to lie down. The Arthritis Foundation and NASA's program on exercise and aging recommend the following flexibility exercises.

For your shoulders:

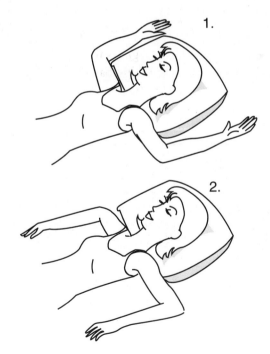

1. Lie on the floor with a pillow under your head, legs straight. If this strains your back, you can place a rolled towel under your knees. Stretch your arms straight out to the side, on the floor. Your upper arms will remain on the floor throughout the exercise. Bend at the elbow so that your hands are pointing toward the ceiling. Let your arms slowly roll backwards from the elbow. Stop when you feel a stretch or slight discomfort. Stop immediately if you feel a pinching sensation or a sharp pain.

2. Slowly raise your arms, still bent at the elbow, toward the ceiling again. Then let your arms slowly roll forward, remaining bent at the elbow, to point toward your hips. Again, stop when you feel a stretch or slight discomfort. Alternate pointing above your head, then toward the ceiling, then toward your hips in this manner. Begin and end with the pointing-above-the-head position. Hold each position for 10 to 30 seconds. Keep your shoulders flat on the floor throughout. Repeat three to five times.

For your hips:

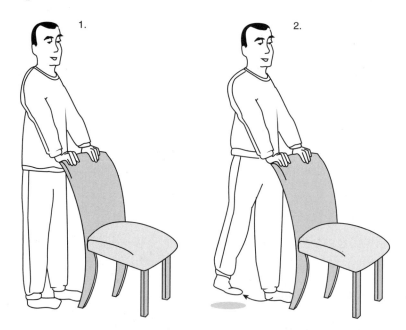

1. Stand erect and hold on to a doorframe or counter or chair back.

2. Move one leg as far out to the side as you can. Keeping your foot stationary, roll your knee in and then out, leading with your heel. Repeat with the other leg.

For your ankles: While seated, flex your foot at the ankle and point your toes. Rotate your foot. Repeat with the other foot.

Yoga and tai chi are excellent for increasing your flexibility, and there are classes available to help you keep to your schedule and stay focused on your goals. Since yoga is so much more than an exercise regimen, you can read about it in greater detail in Chapter 12.

Your local hospital may sponsor one of these programs, or you can contact your YMCA, neighborhood parks and recreation program director, or senior center. You'll find these numbers in your phone book.

Tai chi is an excellent way to get yourself moving and, if you can do this workout outdoors, you'll reap the benefits of fresh air, as well. Tai chi was originally developed in China as a form of self defense, although its graceful movements don't suggest martial arts. It's a gentle form of exercise that you can do at your own pace and comfort level, and you can choose from over 100 movements and positions.

When you have found the positions you want to use, you'll practice them so that one flows into the next without pausing. All of these movements are coordinated with your breathing, so you get the full benefit of stress reduction along with increased flexibility, balance, and stamina. For more information, visit www.taichiforarthritis.com.

Consultation

A 2007 study published in the journal *Arthritis and Rheumatism* found that both hydrotherapy (water therapy) and tai chi for arthritis classes can provide large and sustained improvements in physical function for older, sedentary people with chronic osteoarthritis of the knee or hip.

Strengthening Exercises

Strengthening exercises are also known as resistance exercises. They build the muscles that support your joints. Strong muscles work like shock absorbers, protecting your joints from irritation and injury. The stronger those muscles are, the more protection they can offer. Strengthening exercises use weights or resistance to work the muscles. It's recommended you do them every other day, after your flexibility warm-up. There are two kinds of strengthening exercises: isotonic and isometric. Both of these have good benefits for arthritis.

Isotonic exercises move the joint and involve lengthening (stretching) or shortening (contracting) the muscles associated with that joint. For example, you can extend your leg while you are seated. As you straighten your knee, the joint moves. This exercise strengthens your thigh muscle. Taking the dishes off the counter and placing them in a cupboard above the sink is an isotonic exercise. Walking is also an isotonic exercise, as the muscles in your legs and the muscles associated with your hips both stretch and contract when you take a step.

Isometric exercises do not move the joint. They work by tightening the muscles around the joint. This relieves stress on the joint. For example, to strengthen your back, lie on the floor with knees bent and feet flat on the floor. Tighten your stomach muscles and your buttocks and push the small of your back against the floor. Hold this position for 10 seconds and then relax. This maneuver is called a pelvic tilt. If you are a practitioner of yoga, you are quite familiar with isometric exercise.

To strengthen your hips, grab hold of a doorframe or counter. Move one leg backward and up behind you. Keep your knee straight. Keep your posture straight. Hold for a count of 10 and then release. You should not strength train the same muscle groups on consecutive days. Your muscles need recovery time.

Strengthening or stretching your quadriceps muscles (the muscles in the front of your thighs) is important if you have arthritis. NASA recommends this exercise: Lie on the floor on your left side. Your hips should be lined up so that the right one is directly above the left one. Rest your head on a pillow or your left hand. Bend your right knee, reach back with your right hand, and hold on to your right heel. If you can't reach your heel with your hand, loop a belt over your right foot. Pull slightly (with your hand or with the belt) until the front of your right thigh feels stretched. Hold the position for 10 to 30 seconds. Reverse position and repeat with other leg. Repeat three to five times on each side. If the back of your thigh cramps during this exercise, stretch your leg and try again, more slowly.

Endurance Exercises

Endurance exercise is also known as aerobic or cardiovascular exercise. Low-impact aerobic exercise is appropriate for people with arthritis and includes a wide variety of activities, such as walking outside or on a treadmill, riding a standard or stationary bicycle, or using an elliptical machine. There's bound to be something tailor-made just for you. Try reading a magazine, listening to music, or watching TV while you're on the treadmill or elliptical machine. The time will go by much faster!

Got rhythm? Endurance exercise uses the body's large muscle groups in rhythmic, continuous motions. And yes, that definitely includes dancing! It also includes swimming, bicycling, and golf, among other activities. This form of exercise primes your cardiovascular system to work more efficiently. There are numerous other health benefits, as well, including improved quality of sleep, stronger bones, weight control, and reduced levels of stress, depression, and anxiety.

Too often, the pain of arthritis causes you to reduce the amount of physical activity you do each day. It then becomes a downward spiral. As your joints stiffen even more, you do less and less until any movement at all is painful. Aerobic activity can reverse the damage caused by this sedentary lifestyle.

You'll try for an aerobic activity three to four times a week, with a goal of working at your *target heart rate* for 30 minutes each session. Again, you're going to start slowly—perhaps 5 minutes for starters—and increase gradually as your strength and endurance increase. Don't push yourself. You should be able to hold a conversation while you are exercising. If you are gasping for breath, you're not exercising efficiently. Slow down!

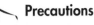

Precautions

High-impact aerobic exercise, such as racquetball, jogging, skiing, football, in-line skating, or step aerobics, increases stress on joints and should be avoided. Use common sense. If you have severe knee arthritis, even a low-impact activity such as riding a bicycle may be too painful. If you have advanced elbow arthritis, you shouldn't use a rowing machine.

def•i•ni•tion

Target heart rate is the term for the optimum pulse rate you reach during exercise, when your circulatory system is working at full efficiency. Check out www.mayoclinic.com/health/target-heart-rate/SM00083 for an easy-to-use target heart rate calculator.

You know that your arthritis is a chronic condition and you also know that exercise is going to help you control that condition. It should be so simple, but human nature, being what it is, makes exercise anything but simple. If you've started an ambitious program before, only to lapse after a couple of weeks, you're among the majority. Fortunately, there are ways around this setback. Stay motivated by …

- Exercising with a friend.

- Finding an activity you really like.

- Building in a reward system for yourself.

Doing your flexibility exercises first thing in the morning can become routine. That's good. In fact, that's wonderful. These exercises seem to be the easiest to remember to do and to do faithfully. The strengthening exercises, while also fairly easy to do, tend to suffer from occasional and not-so-occasional neglect. They take a little more effort and self-discipline. And the aerobic exercises take genuine commitment. It becomes all too easy to postpone them and then, too often, we conveniently forget to do them. Arthritis doesn't forget to give you problems, however, so it really is in your best interest to keep at the program. In this case, easiest is best.

Let's check back with your physical therapist now. You've settled on a regular schedule of exercise and chosen specific activities that will help address your arthritis symptoms. You'll commit to a certain number of sessions with your PT and you'll begin to develop the habit of good exercise. You'll learn to begin each session with a warm-up, and your PT may apply heat at the start of each session, to get blood flowing to the target area.

Straight Talk

"I look forward to my TENS treatment. It means I've successfully completed my physical therapy session. It feels good."

—Jerome, age 45, diagnosed with rheumatoid arthritis at age 32

When you've completed your session, your PT may apply cold packs to the target area. This is designed to reduce inflammation. You may also have an ultrasound or TENS (transcutaneous electrical nerve stimulation) treatment to promote pain relief in your affected joints before you go on your way. A TENS unit is a small device that directs mild electrical impulses to nerves in the painful joint area. These nerve impulses work to block pain signals and may also release endorphins. A TENS treatment may feel like a tingling sensation, but it doesn't hurt.

After you've completed your course of work with your physical therapist, you may want additional support. Perhaps you know your habits and know that you'll have difficulty keeping up your program. If this is you, you may want to take advantage of a new type of exercise specialist, called a clinical exercise specialist. These specialists have additional training and experience to help them work with people with arthritis and other chronic medical conditions.

Hospitals that offer wellness programs may be able to provide you with names of clinical exercise specialists in your area. Their fees may not be covered by your insurance, so check with your carrier. A certified fitness trainer may also have some of this training.

Walking

What's the easiest aerobic activity? It's walking. You can do this one alone or team up with a friend. Make a daily appointment to meet for half an hour and make that walk part of your routine. This may also be the perfect time to get a dog, or if you already have one, to get the leash and take your four-legged walking buddy outside.

Walking is a strengthening exercise for your muscles and bones. Since you're putting your full weight on your bones, this can help prevent osteoporosis, which may be a concern if you're taking corticosteroids for your arthritis symptoms. These medications can weaken your bones.

Walking is also a flexibility exercise, keeping your joints moving to avoid stiffness. As an added benefit, you'll increase your stamina. The Arthritis Foundation can give you information about exercise programs in your area. A 12-week walking plan for beginner, intermediate, and advanced levels is downloadable from the website at www.arthritisfoundation.org. You can also get information there about the Arthritis Walk, the foundation's major fundraiser, which takes place all over the country. See Appendix C for contact information.

Consultation

The life span of a pair of exercise shoes or sneakers is about six months of active use. After that they need to be replaced.

Water Exercise

When your joints are so sore that any impact at all with a firm object sends shock waves throughout your body, water can be a godsend. Water supports your weight, and you will find that movements are much easier in this environment. With less stress on your hips, knees, and spine, you can focus on your exercise program with greater comfort.

In addition, water adds the element of resistance to your movements, and this builds muscle strength. Remember that resistance is not the same thing as impact. Impact stresses joints; resistance strengthens them.

When you immerse your body in warm water, your body temperature rises and causes your blood vessels to dilate and increase blood flow to your joints. This is the equivalent of a warm-up.

The amount of water you have access to will determine the number and types of exercises you can do. Your physical therapy center may have a pool on site for hydrotherapy, but if it doesn't, you can check out your neighborhood community center or YMCA. Other options include a hot tub, spa, or even a simple bathtub. Spas can add the element of massage, with the pulsating release of warm water and air.

If your rheumatologist or physician has prescribed a regimen of water therapy for your arthritis, the cost of a hot tub or spa may be tax deductible as a medical expense. Check with your attorney or accountant for the requirements governing this and be sure to keep all receipts.

Precautions _____

While warm water is beneficial, hot water can be dangerous if you have high blood pressure or coronary artery disease, and it's not necessary. Water temperatures between 83 and 88°F are considered comfortable for exercise. If you feel lightheaded or nauseated, get out of the pool. Also, never consume alcohol before entering the pool, as this can cause drowsiness or changes in blood pressure.

The Arthritis Foundation has an aquatic program specifically designed for people with arthritis and related conditions. This program meets two to three times a week at local indoor pools for 45- to 60-minute sessions with a trained instructor. For more information on the program, contact your local branch of the Arthritis Foundation. While you're at it, ask for their brochure "Water Exercise: Pools, Spas and Arthritis." It's free and packed with good information.

Hand Exercises

If you have rheumatoid arthritis, stiff fingers and pain are unwelcome companions. Following verbal or written instructions for doing hand exercises can be confusing. The Mayo Clinic, however, has an online slide show with clear instructions and photographs of five different hand exercises you can do to increase your strength and flexibility. You can find them at www.mayoclinic.com/health/arthritis/AR00030.

Balancing Rest and Exercise

Balance is important in just about everything, and that includes exercising with arthritis. There are certain times when rest is more important than moving; for example, when you're having a flare. When your joints are hot, swollen, and painful, they need to be rested, not pushed. Talk with your rheumatologist and physical therapist about what kinds of activities are appropriate during flares.

Conserving Energy

When you are tired, you are more prone to injury. This goes for everyone, whether they are dealing with arthritis or not. During flares or during times when you are feeling subpar, take a cue from your body. You need to respect what it is telling you. This does not mean that you give up on your exercise program, but rather that you understand there will be times when you need to modify what you are doing or let your body rest. Taking a short break may be just what your body needs to help it get back on track.

Respecting Pain

You're walking five days a week now and you're generally feeling good about it. You decide to increase your stride and push yourself harder. Two hours after you've finished your walk, however, you're still hurting. You know that you've done too much and pushed too hard. It's fine to be comfortably tired and even a little sore after you've finished exercising, but you shouldn't be hurting an hour after you're done. Shorten your stride, slow down, and you'll still reap the benefits.

Consultation _____

If a cane or walking stick helps you keep on an even keel, use it! Keeping your posture correct will help ward off fatigue and will conserve energy. You won't lose any points for making a smart decision. A walking stick is particularly helpful if you're walking on uneven surfaces or down steep hills or steps. If you're going on a trip where seeing old castles and museums requires more walking than usual, buy a folding walking stick and put it in your suitcase. Many foreign countries may not offer handicapped access.

Recreational Activities and Arthritis

Many recreational activities can provide you with the exercise you need. The key is finding the ones you like and will be likely to keep doing. If you enjoyed a specific kind of recreational activity as a youngster, it may be time to revisit that activity and make the necessary modifications so you can enjoy it once again. For example, if you loved to bicycle as a child, then rediscovering bicycling may be just the ticket to arthritis relief for you.

Sometimes just minor adaptations can enhance your enjoyment of your leisure activities and recreation. While tennis is not a good choice, golf can be—especially if you take the opportunity to walk while on the course. Motorized carts can carry your clubs while you walk alongside. Using lower compression balls will result in more give when you hit the ball and reduce the jarring you experience with impact. You can also build up your grip to allow you to hold the club more easily if you have arthritis in your hands. And always use a tee to avoid the shock that comes when a missed swing results in rearranging the dirt.

If you garden, and millions of Americans do, you can enjoy this activity even if you have arthritis. Do your stretching exercises before you begin to work in the garden. Take breaks while you're out there and stretch during those breaks, as well. Finally, remember to stretch when you're done. Change activities at least every 30 minutes. Take the time to enjoy your garden's beauty. Raised beds can get you off the ground as well. Use the largest muscle group you can for each job. For example, carry items on your forearms instead of grasping them with your hands. Keep good posture all the time. Don't slump! Plan your time, and if you feel yourself getting tired, take a break. Gardening is a process. It's never really done!

Traveling is also a form of leisure activity and recreation. If you have arthritis, it takes a little extra planning, but you can still enjoy the ride. The secret is in planning ahead. Here are some tips for easier traveling:

◆ Don't wait until the last minute to make your reservations. If you need a hotel room that is handicap accessible, be sure it's waiting for you.

◆ When traveling by air, ask for a seat with the most leg room. Give yourself plenty of time if you have to change planes. The bigger airports provide jitney service between terminals, and this will help you conserve your energy.

◆ Request a wheelchair if your arthritis will be aggravated by the kind of walking you'll encounter at the airport.

◆ Take advantage of preboarding opportunities to get yourself settled before the crowds surge onto the plane.

◆ Use valet parking.

◆ Don't overpack, but be sure to bring your prescriptions.

Actually, what works for folks with arthritis also works for everyone else as well. Most of us have a tendency to overpack and we end up hauling around extra pounds of clothes we never wear. A good rule is to pack everything you think you'll need and then return half of it to your closet or dresser!

If you know that you'll be met at the other end of your journey, it's surprising how much more relaxed your travel will be. And with today's technology, you can program essential phone numbers into your phone and have them with you ready for speed dial.

Having arthritis doesn't mean having to give up doing the activities you have always enjoyed. It does mean that you'll be looking for ways to adapt these activities so that you can continue to enjoy them.

The Least You Need to Know

- ◆ Exercise increases flexibility and strength in arthritic joints.
- ◆ Your physical therapist can design a program suited just for you.
- ◆ Flexibility, strength, and endurance exercises are essential components of your exercise program.
- ◆ When you are experiencing a flare, slow down!
- ◆ Recreation should be enjoyable, not an endurance activity.

Chapter 18

Parenting a Child with Juvenile Arthritis

In This Chapter

- Facing the future: communication is essential
- Your rights and responsibilities at school
- How siblings are affected
- Maintaining family routine
- Safeguarding your own health
- Where to turn for help

You want to protect your child from harm, but a diagnosis of a chronic disease, such as juvenile arthritis (JA), can make you feel helpless. You aren't helpless, however, and juvenile arthritis isn't hopeless. Creating as normal a childhood as possible is the greatest gift you can give your child. In this chapter, we'll explore just what that means and how you can accomplish it. (See Chapter 5 for a review of juvenile arthritis.)

After the Diagnosis

Receiving a diagnosis of a chronic condition is difficult enough to absorb when it concerns you. It's much more difficult to deal with when it concerns your child. A child's illness is a parent's greatest fear, but you can take solace in the fact that there's a very good chance your child will come out of the experience without permanent effects. While you're waiting for that positive outcome, you're going to have questions, and you're going to need answers.

Coming to Grips

There are certain predictable stages we pass through when faced with life-changing situations. Dr. Elisabeth Kübler-Ross documented these as denial, anger, bargaining, resignation, and acceptance. You'll undoubtedly pass through each of these stages after you learn your child has JA:

1. **Denial.** "What? How is this possible? There must be a mistake." Your first reaction may be one of disbelief. You took your child to the doctor because she was limping or because her knee was swollen. You were expecting a simple diagnosis with a quick resolution.

2. **Anger.** "Why my child? This isn't fair." You can't protect your child and so you feel angry. It's a normal reaction.

3. **Bargaining.** "Surely there's something we can do? What if she just rests for a bit?" You're beginning to understand this is a serious matter, but the scope is beyond your experience.

4. **Resignation.** "All right. I understand. I didn't do anything to cause this. This is just one of those things that happens. I guess it could be worse."

5. **Acceptance.** "So, what do we do? What's the first step? What's the prognosis? Let's get moving."

All of these stages may pass very quickly, often within an initial office visit. As a parent, you're used to rolling with the punches, but this is a serious hit. It will take a little time to get your bearings and regain your balance.

Your immediate next step will depend in large part upon the age of your child and the type of JA he has. It's fairly easy to bundle up a toddler and head back home. You're driving, your head is spinning, but your child is in the car seat in the back and you've got a little time to sort things through.

If your child is old enough to understand that something is wrong, you may not have that buffer time to pull yourself together. The child's questions may come immediately. What you say in those first few moments can set the stage for growth for everyone in the family.

Consultation

Elisabeth Kübler-Ross, author of the landmark book *On Death and Dying* (Scribner, 1997), was a medical doctor who spent her lifetime learning about how people approached death, dying, and transitional change in their lives.

First Things First

The most important thing you can do for your child, your family, and yourself is to maintain a positive outlook. This can be incredibly difficult when you are worried and uncertain about what the future holds. However, your child will look to you for clues to how to react. Your child will view JA the same way you do, so projecting positivity and reassurance is essential. If that means smiling while you're fighting back tears, that's just what you'll do.

Making an association with another medical condition that has a good prognosis is a positive way to start explaining JA to a child. If you know of another child with a chronic condition, such as asthma, for example, who is doing well with medication and regular doctor appointments, this could be a good choice. You want to reduce your child's anxiety level, and by making this sort of association, you'll reduce your own, as well.

Talking Is Important

Once you're back home, your child will have questions, just as you do. Answer them in a matter-of-fact tone. You don't have to know all the answers, but listening to and validating your child's concerns are vital. Honesty is essential to building trust. That works for adults and it works for children. Your child will know if you're holding back or not telling the truth. And rather than building trust, this creates fear.

"I don't know the answer to that question, honey; let's write it down in your journal and we'll ask the doctor," is a fine answer to a child's question. If your child is old enough to write, have her keep track of her questions under your supervision.

Don't be surprised when your child expresses anger. This is a natural reaction. Your child can be frustrated by the limits JA places on him and needs to know that you understand this. Trust your instincts. If you become concerned that your child's anger isn't improving, talk to your doctor to see if your child might benefit from counseling. Your rheumatologist, nurse specialist, or social worker will be able to help you find the best resources.

Guilt is another feeling your child may experience. Young children may believe that they have been bad and that getting sick is punishment for their bad behavior. This may sound foolish to you, but it can be very real to your child. Tell your child that this illness isn't his fault; it's nobody's fault. Sometimes people get sick, and you're going to do everything you can to help him get better.

> **Precautions**
>
> Answer specific questions as they come up, but resist the impulse to launch into an extensive explanation of your child's condition. Your child can only process a little information at a time.

Your other children will also have questions. They may wonder if JA is contagious, if life will ever return to "normal," and what is going to be expected of them. Answer them honestly. If you don't know, say so. If you do, tell them.

You will need to talk about your concerns, as well. Learning to cope involves much more than just getting through the day. It means becoming actively engaged in a host of problem-solving activities. If you have been a "go it alone" or "do it yourself" kind of person, it's time to ask for some help. Family and friends are there for you.

Encouraging Independence

Your natural reaction may be to protect your child from additional harm. This can backfire if you allow your protective instincts to overshadow your common sense and parenting skills. Allow your child as much freedom and responsibility as possible in completing chores, participating in family activities, and doing things for himself. When you must alter your child's activities, however, offer a compromise activity that will support your child's independence. JA is not an excuse to withdraw from life.

Encourage your child to read about his condition and what he can expect. The fear of the unknown is the greatest worry. When your child is experiencing a flare-up, he may be more tired and irritable and have difficulty concentrating. Be sure he gets the rest he needs: "You can clean up your room tomorrow, when you're feeling better."

Give your child choices whenever possible. Many children with a chronic disease feel as if they don't have control over anything. They certainly don't have control over their bodies, they reason, so they can feel powerless. Having choices also builds independence and has the added benefit of often preventing conflict: "Would you rather have spaghetti or hamburgers tonight?" "Do you want to swim today or ride your bicycle?"

When it's appropriate, extend these choices to medical matters. At home, if your child is old enough, give him the responsibility for choosing which pain picture on the pain scale should go into the journal for that day. At the doctor's office, ask, "Which arm is better for getting your shot today?"

Chores and Responsibilities

Giving your child responsibilities tells her that she is an important member of the family. Being trusted with certain chores and responsibilities builds character and confidence. It also reinforces for the child that she isn't different from other children. Feeding the cat or dog and changing the water in the bowl, setting or clearing the table, or other chores that your child can do will encourage your child to grow up to be a responsible adult.

Keep your daily routines as much as you can. There will be times when medical appointments or other unexpected events disrupt your daily schedule, but if you keep routines in place, your child will feel more secure and won't think that her JA is controlling everyone's lives.

Discipline

All children misbehave. It doesn't matter whether they have a chronic illness or not. Don't be afraid to discipline your child. Setting limits and establishing consequences for when a child goes beyond those limits builds confidence, security, trust, and a sense of being loved.

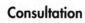

Consultation _____

Children instinctively look for limits and keep pushing until they find them. Limits offer security. A child who has no limits never learns right from wrong.

Praise your child when she does her chores and discipline her when she doesn't. Of course, when your child is experiencing a flare or is ill, you'll modify your expectations. You'd do that anyway with any child who was ill.

Be consistent in your discipline, and your child will understand what's allowed and what isn't. She also won't learn to use her illness as an excuse for not living a healthy and productive life. Time-outs for young children and restricting privileges for older ones work whether your child is healthy or dealing with a chronic illness.

Dealing with Hurts

If your child is wearing a brace or if her joints are noticeably swollen, she may feel that everyone is looking at her. This is an opportunity to help prepare her for occasions when someone may stare or make a rude or insensitive comment. Being matter-of-fact is the best way to deal with the situation.

Teasing is a normal but disturbing part of childhood, and every child is vulnerable to this kind of bullying. The same techniques you would use to help your child face a bully if she didn't have JA also apply here. How you approach this teaching opportunity will depend on your child's age and personality. A self-confident child might not need much help beyond the knowledge that you're behind him, supporting him.

If your child needs more help, you can give it. If the problem is happening with a playmate, talk to that child's parents about what's happening. It's important not to be threatening, but rather to go seeking their help. If bullying is happening at school, talk to your child's teacher. Bullying at school often happens outside the classroom, in the halls or at recess, away from the eyes and ears of the teacher, so he may not be aware of the problem. If talking to the teacher doesn't help, go to the principal with your concerns. Don't stop until you've gotten the help you need.

Consultation _____

The old saying "sticks and stones may break my bones, but names can never hurt me" is simply not true. Names do hurt. If your child is being teased, you need to take appropriate action. Scars from childhood hurts can last into adulthood.

Adults may be curious, but they can also be insensitive. It's not uncommon for someone to speak as if your child isn't there and can't hear what's being said. Again, this is your opportunity to educate: "Ashley is right here. Would you like her to explain juvenile arthritis to you?" Often a comment like that is all it takes to get an otherwise compassionate adult to realize what she's done.

At the other end of the insensitive scale is the friend, relative, acquaintance, or total stranger who wants to give you all the benefit of his advice, even if he's never had any experience with juvenile arthritis.

You can try a simple, "Thanks for your concern, but we're following our doctor's advice" and then change the subject immediately to something totally unrelated. If this doesn't work the first time, repeat as often as necessary.

Discussions at home between you and your partner also need to take into account that your child might be listening. If you're not in agreement about medications, the course of treatment, or other issues involving your child, keep your discussions private. Your child needs to see both of you as a united front. Arguing openly will build fear and insecurity.

Preparing for Medical Procedures

When your child is scheduled for a medical appointment that may involve blood tests or preparation for surgery, it's important that she know what to expect. If your child is old enough to worry, she's old enough to know the truth. You may think you're protecting her from unnecessary worry, but the consequences of not preparing her can backfire on you.

If other appointments have been general in nature, and this one is an exception, not preparing her and then having her be surprised may change the way she feels about every appointment from then on. By explaining that this one will be a little different and telling her what will happen, you're keeping her trust.

School Concerns

School is so much more than reading, writing, math, and taking tests. It's the place your child learns important social skills about getting along with other people. Solving problems, resolving disputes, learning independence, and exploring the world of future careers are only small parts of what goes on in your child's daily life at school. It's a complex place, and teachers speak a professional language that may be confusing. As a parent, you have both rights and responsibilities regarding your child's schooling and health-care needs.

Your Rights

Under the Individuals with Disabilities Education Act (IDEA) or the Education for All Handicapped Children Act of 1975, your child is entitled to a free, appropriate public school education in the least restrictive environment appropriate to her needs. This means that the school cannot discriminate against your child because she has a disability—even if that disability is not always evident, as can be the case with JA.

If your child needs special equipment to perform routine classroom tasks or needs an adaptive physical education program, her school is required to make reasonable accommodations for her. This may mean that she dictates her answers on a test to an aide who writes them down for her. It may mean that instead of doing pushups in the gym, she does an alternative exercise that is compatible with her treatment protocol. In cases where an adapted program is necessary, you may be invited to participate in developing an *Individualized Education Program (IEP)* for your child.

def•i•ni•tion

An **Individualized Education Program (IEP)** meeting consists of your child's teachers, the school counselor, the special education teacher, yourself, and your child, if appropriate. During the IEP meeting, all of you will work together to create a coordinated plan to ensure your child's success in school.

Your Responsibilities

Your teachers have your child's best interests at heart. And while they may not know what JA is or how it affects your child, they will be eager to learn what you have to tell them. If your child does not exhibit any observable outward symptoms, her teacher may expect her to perform the same as the other children. It's vitally important to establish good lines of communication early on. Be pleasant, be approachable, and be prepared. Here's a handy list of what to do:

♦ Make an appointment to speak with the principal of your child's school to explain your child's health issues. Bring a letter from your rheumatologist and literature from the Arthritis Foundation to share.

♦ Meet with your child's teachers and explain what they can expect. Ask to be informed if they observe anything out of the ordinary.

♦ If your child will be taking medication while at school, be sure this is given to the proper office personnel for safekeeping.

Being proactive is the best way of preventing problems later on. Enlisting support and building a team approach to helping your child succeed in school is good parenting!

Recreation and Sports

Recreation is not a substitute for physical therapy and therapeutic exercise, but it is an important part of your child's daily life and can complement her treatment plan. Using the lessons learned in physical therapy will help your child avoid injury. Getting out of the house and remaining involved in the normal activities of childhood is essential for your child's physical and emotional health.

Your child may not be able to participate in some much-loved activities right now, but keeping a positive focus on activities your child *can* do will open new windows of opportunity. Consider a summer camp geared to children with JA. Not only will it provide recreation and exercise, but it will also expand your child's network of friends and peers who understand what she is going through.

When a child has a chronic illness or a disability, it's easy for him to think of himself as different or weird. Being in the company of other children with the same disability removes this label and allows your child to just be a kid. It's always easier to be yourself when you're in the company of those who understand how you feel. Children are no different from adults in this regard.

Sibling Relationships

Your other children are also affected by their sibling's diagnosis of JA and will respond and react according to their ages, maturity levels, and personality types. Younger children may withdraw or become clingy, needing constant reassurance that they are healthy and that you still love them. Young children may believe they have caused their sibling to develop JA because they were angry at her.

Older children may react with anger, but this anger is generated by fear. They may fear losing their own health and losing your time and attention. Guilt may also enter the picture. Initial outbursts of anger may

Precautions

Some children feel the need to excel at all kinds of new activities to somehow "make up for" their sibling's loss of mobility. If you notice changes in your other children's behavior, talk with them about their feelings and then suggest appropriate ways they can help out.

dissolve into tears or repressed feelings of guilt about feeling angry. Older children may also show a tendency to overprotect their sibling with juvenile arthritis.

Whether you observe anger, frustration, guilt, or overprotectiveness, understand that these are the ways your children are trying to cope with something they do not understand. Joining with other families who have children with JA can give your other children opportunities to discuss these feelings with their peers. The Arthritis Foundation (www.arthritis.org) has excellent resources for this. Counseling is another option to give your children strategies for managing their feelings. Ask your physician for a referral.

Emotional, Physical, and Financial Concerns

Learning to adjust to new challenges in parenting can cause strain in many aspects of your life. Routines are disrupted, finances become an issue, and fatigue can rob you of your energy.

Stress and anxiety can also lead to feelings of depression. If you find that your energy levels have dropped significantly, that you are struggling to get through the day, or that your eating and sleeping habits have changed, you may be experiencing depression. If these symptoms continue for more than two weeks, check with your doctor. There are effective treatments for depression.

Time and Money

Time becomes a major factor when you're trying to get everything that needs doing done. With your days already scheduled to the max, you must now find the time to provide extra care for your child. This may mean getting up earlier to assist with dressing and hygiene or driving your child to doctor or therapy appointments. It also may mean foregoing some of your usual activities for the present.

Sit down with your family and set up a daily schedule. Eliminate the nonessentials and focus on getting the necessary jobs done.

Ask for help from friends and family members. That's what they're there for. Everyone likes to feel needed, and this is a golden opportunity to let someone else take over some errands or responsibilities until your lives even out again.

Medical care is expensive, even with insurance. You may need to work some overtime, but also need to request time off to attend to health-care matters for your child. How your employer accommodates your needs can make a world of difference to both you and your family. Here again, communication is essential. You'll need to be clear about what you will and won't be able to do for the time being. Your employer will also have concerns about your ability to keep up your previous level of performance. Direct and open discussion can allay those concerns and also enlist your employer's support.

Consultation

Some companies allow employees to pool their unused sick days so that an employee can draw from the sick pool in an emergency. Check to see if this is true of your place of employment. If your company has a union representative or ombudsperson, consider using his services.

A Word About Fatigue

Stress builds when you become physically and emotionally exhausted. Worry about finances, along with wondering about a prognosis for your child, can take its toll on your own well-being. For the sake of your health and that of your family, take time for relaxation and recreation. This is not a luxury—it's essential. You need some alone time, as well as time with friends. This will help to recharge your batteries.

Walking costs nothing, but you'll reap health benefits from a brisk morning or evening walk. Yoga or tai chi also promotes relaxation and rejuvenation. Meditation is another healthful practice that will give you the energy you need to cope.

When you exercise as part of your daily routine, you will sleep better at night. With a good night's rest, you'll be more able to meet the next day's challenges.

See Chapter 15 for more on what you can do to fight fatigue and stay energized.

Worry

Men and women process worry in different ways. Women, in general, tend to reach out when in need of emotional support. Men tend not to.

Often it is Mom who takes the child to doctor appointments and oversees daily medication management and nutrition. These aspects of providing what your child needs can also help you cope with parenting a child with a chronic illness. A familiarity comes with routines and it's important that Dad also have a hand in these aspects of parenting.

A 2004 study took a look at the experience of fathers who had a child with juvenile arthritis. During interviews with 22 dads, researchers found that fathers experienced many emotions as they sought to find effective ways to parent their children. They generally turned inward and, during periods of high stress, overrelied upon self-support strategies to cope. The researchers called upon health-care practitioners to focus greater attention on helping fathers adapt. The study was reported in *Qualitative Health Research.*

Parenting is a partnership. It's easier when both parents are involved in supporting their child and each other. Sharing the load makes it more manageable.

Eating Right: A Family Concern

When your child is hurting, she may not have her usual healthy appetite and she may pick at her food. This usually happens during a flare. Encourage her to eat at meal-time and offer colorful, healthy snacks to tempt her appetite. By serving nutrient-rich foods, you may be able to reduce the amount she needs to eat to maintain optimal growth and nutrition.

You will be tired—both physically and emotionally. At these times, the temptation to rely on fast food can be great. If your child has special dietary requirements, a dietician can show you how to manage them. A dietician can help you plan simple, nutritious, and tasty meals to keep both your and your child's health optimal. Check with your local hospital to find a dietician or ask your rheumatologist for a recommendation.

There is no specific diet for juvenile arthritis. Good nutrition is good nutrition, pure and simple. (See Chapter 16 for more on nutrition basics.) Be sure to include foods rich in calcium in your child's diet, as active JA has been linked to a condition called osteopenia, which may lead to osteoporosis or thinning bones. Getting at least three servings of calcium-rich foods every day can help promote bone health.

Research and Resources

Research into the causes and treatment of juvenile arthritis is ongoing. Current studies are investigating the role that stem cell transplants may play in treating JA. In 1994, the National Institute of Arthritis and Musculoskeletal and Skin Diseases (NIAMS) created a registry for families who have two or more siblings with JA. This will serve as a resource for researchers.

NIAMS is the funding agency for the Multipurpose Arthritis and Musculoskeletal Diseases Center (MAMDC), which specializes in research on pediatric rheumatic diseases, including JA. NIAMS is one of the research institutes of the National Institutes of Health (NIH).

This ongoing registry is updated periodically and is housed at the Children's Hospital Medical Center at the University of Cincinnati College of Medicine. The website for NIAMS is www.niams.nih.gov. The NIH also provides information on clinical trials involving JA. To see if your child qualifies for participation in one of these trials, go to the website www.clinicaltrials.gov.

Your first and best resource is the Arthritis Foundation. If you're looking to connect with other families who have children with JA, this is the place. The Arthritis Foundation sponsors an annual National Juvenile Arthritis Family Conference, along with a national Advocacy and Kids' Summit in Washington, D.C. The Arthritis Foundation is also a source of funding for research into JA. It's led by a JA Council of parents, young adults, pediatric rheumatologists, and advocates who help guide the Arthritis Foundation's approach toward JA.

The Least You Need to Know

- ◆ Open and honest communication with your child will reduce fear and build trust.

- ◆ Treat your child with JA as normally as possible.

- ◆ Your child should attend school and participate in recreational activities as much as she can.

- ◆ Take time to rest and restore your own energy.

- ◆ The Arthritis Foundation is an excellent resource for children with JA and their families.

Chapter 19

Workplace Issues

In This Chapter

- Rethinking your work routine
- Necessary modifications
- Your rights and responsibilities as an employee
- Filing for benefits
- A wealth of information from the Job Accommodation Network (JAN)
- Changing directions

For eight hours a day, and possibly more, you're at work. Work is a source of personal fulfillment, income, and often—stress. Arthritis may well impact your ability to do your job. Sometimes simple modifications are all that it takes to keep you in the game, but at other times you may need the protection of the Americans with Disabilities Act (ADA).

Rethinking the Workplace

Conserving your energy is a primary concern when you have arthritis. This means finding easier ways to accomplish your daily tasks, whether at home or at work. You do so much each day that streamlining your work life may seem too big a task to tackle. Perhaps the easiest way to do it is to sit down and look at the big picture. Think macro before you go micro.

Map out your daily schedule and tasks and then look for assistive devices or techniques to help you get the job done. Where to start? Begin your survey with your wake-up time in the morning. Since it may take you longer to get ready for the daily grind, it makes sense to set your alarm half an hour earlier so you won't be rushed and arrive at work already fatigued. Simple solution for your first task of the day. Mapping out the rest of the day can be just as easy, if you take it one step at a time.

The Daily Commute

Sometimes adaptation can result in unexpected benefits. If you've been a single-passenger car commuter, investigate some alternatives. Many metropolitan areas have vanpools, as well as good transit systems. Perhaps a neighbor who works in the same area or who travels along the same route as you would like to carpool. Once you begin looking at ways to ease your commute, you'll see options you didn't know were there. Giving up the solitary commute, if it's a viable option, has many benefits:

- Lower monthly gas bills
- Less wear and tear on your car
- Savings on parking costs
- Time to read or listen to music
- Less stress

Sharing your ride is also the environmentally friendly thing to do, and it lets you breeze along in the carpool lane while others are stuck in traffic.

If you have to drive yourself, there are adaptive devices made for your car. Knobs, grips, and steering cuffs eliminate the need to grip the steering wheel if your hands are affected with arthritis. You'll find a selection of these devices on the Job Accommodation Network (JAN) website, www.jan.wvu.edu. (We discuss the Job Accommodation Network later in this chapter.)

Modifying Your Work Environment

Once at work, take a critical look at your surroundings. Before you go to your supervisor and explain that your cubicle, desk, office, or physical environment isn't going to cut it anymore, look for changes you can make on your own. Can you adjust your chair for more comfort? Can you rearrange your workspace to make it more efficient and create fewer demands on your joints? Look at your desk, for example. Are your hole punch, stapler, and phone within easy reach or do you have to bend, stretch, or otherwise contort yourself to reach them?

Your goals are to protect your joints and to prevent fatigue, and this is where an occupational therapist (OT) can help you. Your rheumatologist can refer you to an OT, who will show you how to make additional changes to help you get through the workday more easily.

Consultation _____

Be kind to your feet. If you're a slave to fashion, your feet are going to hurt. Wear athletic shoes to and from work and change into a pair of comfortable dress shoes on the job. Women, remember that narrow toes and stiletto heels are bad for your back, your joints, your arthritis, and your comfort.

If you don't have an ergonomic keyboard for your computer and a gel pad to support your wrist while using your mouse, these would be good investments. They won't break the office budget, but even if you have to spring for them on your own, you'll be doing your joints a favor. You'll also be more prepared when it's time to talk to your supervisor, having already taken the initiative to make some necessary changes.

Rate of Output

Whatever your job, the bottom line for your employer is results. Whether you're paid by the piece, by the hour, on commission, or on salary, your output determines company profits and company profits determine your job security. If your productivity declines because you're not able to work at the same pace or at the same level you did before arthritis entered the picture, you can expect to hear about it in one way or another.

If your work requires a high level of physical activity, you'll be more impacted by arthritis than someone who is more sedentary at work. However, all work involves some physical activity. Standing or sitting for extended periods of time can result in stiffness and difficulty in performing tasks. Change your position frequently to avoid stiffening up.

Arthritis isn't predictable. Flares can come at the most inconvenient times, and if you're fatigued and hurting, you're not going to be able to pretend you're not. Fortunately, you have options, and one of them is the Americans with Disabilities Act.

Arthritis and Disability

The Americans with Disabilities Act (ADA) was passed by Congress in 1990 and went into effect July 26, 1992. The law prohibits private employers with 15 or more employees, state and local governments, employment unions, and labor unions from discriminating against qualified individuals with disabilities in job application procedures, hiring, firing, advancement, compensation, and job training and in other terms, conditions, and privileges of employment.

According to the ADA, employers are required to make a reasonable accommodation to those with a known *disability*, as long as that accommodation does not create an undue hardship on the operation of that business.

def•i•ni•tion

The Americans with Disabilities Act defines a **disability** as a physical or mental impairment that substantially limits one or more of the major life activities of such individual, a record of such an impairment, or being regarded as having such an impairment.

The ADA does not contain a list of medical conditions that qualify as disabilities. Instead, the ADA has a general definition of disability that each person must meet. Therefore, some people with arthritis will be considered to have a disability under the ADA and some will not.

What does "reasonable accommodation" mean? If you would be able to continue at your job if your work schedule were modified, your job were restructured, you were moved to half- or part-time, or you were reassigned to a vacant position, then your employer is obligated to make those changes at no cost to you.

With the dawn of the information age, the nature of work in many fields has been restructured. Flex time, working from home (telecommuting), job sharing, and a host of other inventive approaches to the workplace have become more common. Unfortunately, outsourcing and downsizing have also become commonplace, and job security can no longer be taken for granted. And there will always be jobs where these creative approaches to managing work time don't apply. On the one hand, it's become easier to manage work if you have a disability; on the other, it's become more complicated.

Your Responsibilities as an Employee

If you want to be covered under the Americans with Disabilities Act, your employer needs to know about your medical condition. You've got to disclose. Depending upon the severity of your arthritis, you may consider applying for disability benefits, requesting reasonable accommodations at work, or choosing to tough it out and see if you can make do with the situation as it is. Communication with your employer is essential if your performance on the job has been or will be affected by your arthritis.

If your pain is severe or if you are experiencing flares, it will become apparent to your co-workers and your supervisor that you are not producing up to standards. Denial on your part won't change the reality. So, how much to disclose? This will depend upon several factors:

- Your position within your company

- The security of your position

- The severity of your arthritis

- Your potential need for time off work

- Your relationship with your supervisor

You can't be productive if you're operating in a climate of fear. If you've been prescribed splints to help support your joints, for example, and you aren't wearing them because you're concerned they make you appear weak or not up to the job, then you're not doing what's best to manage your arthritis. The truth will probably come out eventually. If you're in pain, you're not going to be at the top of your game, and, splints or not, co-workers and supervisors will notice.

"Last hired, first fired" is an all too familiar workplace saying. Unfortunately, if you fall into this category, you may feel the need to conceal your arthritis in order to keep your job. During a flare, you may or may not be able to pull this off.

Only you can make this decision. It all revolves around what kind of work you do. If your job places physical demands on your body, such as lifting, carrying, kneeling, standing, or considerable walking, you may find that you have great difficulty getting through the day and that ultimately you may not be able to continue at that particular job. If your work is dictated by a rigid schedule, you also may not be able to keep with it, especially during flares or when fatigue has sapped your energy.

If you find yourself using sick days more frequently than you used to or are having difficulty getting to work on time, management may get the idea that you're unreliable, which is the first step toward termination. Addressing your health issues up front and honestly may prevent this from happening.

Sick Leave and Job Loss

A 2007 study appearing in the *International Archives of Occupational and Environmental Health* looked at the role of sick leave as a risk factor for job loss. It followed 112 people with chronic arthritis and a disease-related problem at work. Researchers defined "sick leave" as absenteeism reported to the employer and "job loss" as receiving a full work disability pension or unemployment. After 24 months, 23 percent of the participants in the study had lost their jobs. The researchers also found that anxiety and depression were significantly associated with this job loss at a two-year follow-up.

Precautions

In a competitive job market, reaching age 50 can make it difficult to get a job and difficult to keep one. The incidence of rheumatic disease rises with age, and onset of a rheumatic disease can make your job situation even more precarious. Know your rights under the law.

Using up all your sick leave and hoping to keep your job don't appear to be compatible. Becoming proactive in managing both your health care and your employment is a better choice.

Vocational Rehabilitation

Losing your job involves much more than loss of a paycheck. Research has shown that for individuals with rheumatic diseases, job loss also involves higher levels of depression and pain. Losing your job due to health-related issues is associated with loss of self-esteem, life satisfaction, and personal perceptions of health status. Coming to grips with a chronic health condition means taking steps to safeguard your job and your financial future.

The National Institute of Arthritis and Musculoskeletal and Skin Diseases sponsored research that looked at how vocational rehabilitation might improve job retention for patients with rheumatic diseases. The four-year study begun in 2000 followed 242 individuals with rheumatic diseases who had said they were at risk for job loss. The study participants were assigned to two groups. One group received three hours of vocational rehabilitation services focusing on job accommodation, vocational counseling, education, and self-advocacy. The other group was given printed materials about disability employment issues and resources through the mail. The study found that vocational rehabilitation reduced job loss by 49 percent compared to those who didn't receive this intervention.

The Rehabilitation Services Administration (RSA) is the federal agency overseeing vocational rehabilitation programs, counseling, medical and psychological services, job training, supported employment, and independent living services. The RSA funds programs in every state. The RSA website is www.ed.gov/about/offices/list/osers/rsa/index.html

Applying for Benefits

If you find you are unable to work because of arthritis, you may be eligible for Social Security benefits. Each case is decided on an individual basis by the Social Security Administration. You will need specific information and complete medical records in order to complete the application for disability benefits.

Two Social Security programs provide disability benefits: Supplemental Security Income (SSI) and Social Security Disability Insurance (SSDI). Medical qualifying requirements are the same for both programs, and disability is determined by the same process for both programs. To begin the process of applying for benefits, you can do one of the following:

- Go to www.ssa.gov/applyfordisability to complete an online application.

- Call Social Security's toll-free number: 1-800-772-1213.

- Call SSI's hearing-impaired number: TTY 1-800-325-0778.

- Call or visit your local Social Security office. The address and phone number will be in the government section of your local telephone directory.

Precautions

Two of every three applications for benefits are initially denied. If you are denied benefits, you may petition for a review of that decision. Applications for disability take longer than other Social Security procedures. The process may take from three to five months.

Social Security provides a Disability Planner that gives specific information on the process of applying for benefits.

To apply, you will need the following materials:

- Your Social Security number and proof of your age

- Names, addresses, and phone numbers of doctors, case workers, hospitals, and clinics that provided services to you, along with the dates of your appointments

- Names and dosages of all your medications

- Laboratory and test results

- All medical records pertaining to your condition

- A summary of where you worked and the kind of work you did

- Your most recent W-2 form, or, if you were self-employed, a copy of your federal tax return

If you aren't successful in obtaining Social Security benefits, you have other options that may help you keep your job.

Job Accommodation Network

The Job Accommodation Network (JAN) is a free service of the Office of Disability Employment Policy (ODEP) of the United States Department of Labor. Its mission is to facilitate the employment and retention of workers with disabilities by providing employers, employment providers, people with disabilities, their family members, and other interested parties with information on job *accommodations*, self-employment and small business opportunities, and related subjects. Numerous resources are available through the JAN website, www.jan.wvu.edu.

def•i•ni•tion

An **accommodation** is any modification or adjustment to a job, work environment, or the way things are usually done that enables a qualified individual with a disability to enjoy an equal employment opportunity.

JAN provides a wealth of information. If you have had difficulty locating resources pertaining to your employment, it is the place to visit. It's also the place to learn what reasonable accommodations might be and how they can fit into your specific work situation. Check out their publication "Accommodation and Compliance Series: Employees with Arthritis." See Appendix C for contact information.

Some of the solutions JAN proposes are not only appropriate for people with arthritis, but also make sense for employees without any disabling medical condition. Flexible work hours, frequent or extended breaks, working from home, and implementing ergonomic workstation designs are among the accommodations that can be termed "reasonable." Other accommodations include ...

- A scooter or other mobility aid if walking cannot be reduced.

- Writing and grip aids.

- A page turner and book holder.

- Providing parking close to the work site.

- Speech recognition software.

- A stand/lean stool for jobs that require prolonged standing.

JAN also provides vendor lists for various accommodation products and will direct you to the appropriate supplier for your specific needs.

If you've been reluctant to request accommodations because you think the cost of accommodating your needs will be too high, don't be! A recent study of employers who used the Job Accommodation Network found that more than half of the accommodations needed by employees and job applicants cost absolutely nothing. Of the ones that did incur a cost, the average expenditure was about $600. Examples of no-cost accommodations include changing a work schedule or assigning a parking space close to the entrance.

Accommodations provided indirect benefits to employers, as well. They reported that company production increased overall, morale was improved throughout the company, a valued employee could be retained, the costs of training a new employee were eliminated, and, most importantly, the accommodation increased the productivity of the employee with the disability.

> **Straight Talk**
>
> I couldn't grip a pen. I found out that I could push my pen through a Styrofoam ball and grip the ball, using gross motor movements instead of small motor movements to write. What a difference!
>
> —Laine, age 23, diagnosed with rheumatoid arthritis in her hands

Changing Employers

The time may come when you decide to change jobs. Perhaps you are re-entering the workplace after a long-term absence, or perhaps this is your first venture into the world of work. Whatever your situation, there are some special challenges you will face when you have arthritis.

> **Precautions**
>
> When do you disclose your medical condition? The time to do this is after you have been offered the job and have accepted it. If you can perform your job duties with reasonable accommodation, you cannot be fired because of your disability.

If you will need additional time at lunch to rest or if you'll need time off for doctor appointments or medical procedures, provide a plan for making up that time. Your employer will be more willing to accommodate you if you are willing to accommodate your employer.

Under the provisions of the ADA, your employer cannot charge you for the cost of accommodations to your workplace. If the cost will create an undue hardship for your employer, you must be given the choice of assuming the cost on your own or of sharing the cost.

The purpose of the law is to help you remain employed. However, if you feel you have been discriminated against because of your arthritis, you can file a complaint with the Equal Employment Opportunity Commission (EEOC) and other federal agencies. A complaint should be a last resort, and other means of resolving the problem, such as negotiation, mediation, and arbitration make more financial sense for both you and your employer.

If you do file a formal complaint, this should be done within 180 days of the time the discrimination occurred. Ask your employer for copies of all letters and reports relating to the situation. If your complaint is upheld, you are entitled to a remedy that will place you in the position you would have been in if the discrimination hadn't happened. You may be entitled to hiring, promotion, reinstatement, back pay, attorney's fees, or reasonable accommodation—which may include reassignment to a different job.

Family and Medical Leave Act (FMLA)

The Family and Medical Leave Act (FMLA) went into effect in August 1993. This Act provides for employees who need to take up to 12 weeks of unpaid medical leave per year if a serious health condition prevents them from working. Working part-time, taking installments, or taking the entire 12 weeks at once is permitted. This Act applies to companies with more than 50 employees.

To be eligible, you must have worked for your employer for 1,250 hours in the previous 12 months.

You cannot be denied your rights under this Act, and your workplace is required to post a notice of your rights under the FMLA.

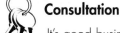

Consultation

It's good business and good manners to give your employer as much advance notice as you can if you'll need to take an unpaid leave. This allows time to find a temporary replacement for you and ensure a smooth transition. It also keeps communication avenues open, an essential part of doing business.

Getting Real

In an ideal world, there would be no repercussions for disclosing a disability at work. The reality is, however, that discrimination can occur, and it can be subtle. Proving you have been discriminated against can be difficult. Did you not get that promotion because you disclosed your disability or because someone else was truly more qualified? Even when objective criteria are used to assess job performance, there's always an element of subjectivity in the picture.

It's essential that you keep accurate records of your output and work performance. This can become tedious, especially when your arthritis is causing you fatigue and pain. But if you believe that you have been the victim of discrimination on the job, this record of accomplishment will become important.

If your work atmosphere is congenial and supportive, you'll find your job is that much easier to accomplish. If the atmosphere is strained or hostile, however, and if you believe you cannot trust your supervisor or one or more of your co-workers, your job will tax your energy and strength. You may decide it's time to explore your options.

Whether you're a telecommuter or an entrepreneur, there are distinct advantages to working from home. Of course, there are also some drawbacks. If you're finding it difficult to handle the commute and the rigid structure of the workplace, however, working from home may be a good choice.

The Small Business Administration (SBA) offers a Handicapped Assistance Loan program (HAL-2) that provides direct loans and loan guarantees to qualified individuals with disabilities who wish to start their own businesses. The SBA can also offer individual guidance and classes for people who are starting up their own business. You can also find classes online and at local community and adult education programs.

Working at home can be both financially rewarding and personally fulfilling. It requires self-discipline to spend the amount of time required to make your job successful. Keeping focused on work during the workday is essential. This means being able to tune out distractions that are more common at home than in a traditional work setting.

One of the most common complaints of those working at home is interruptions by family members who don't recognize that you're working. From the beginning, make it clear to your loved ones that when your door is closed, you are working and aren't available unless the house is burning down. Once your family has gotten the message, working at home can help you pace yourself and conserve your energy while still remaining productive.

Whether you remain employed in the traditional workplace or explore the new frontier of working from home, arthritis does not have to be the deciding or the limiting factor in that choice.

The Least You Need to Know

- Modifying your work environment will help you remain productive on the job.
- The Americans with Disabilities Act provides you with legal recourse should you lose your job because of a medical disability.
- Social Security provides benefits for individuals with medical disabilities, but the requirements are stringent.
- The Job Accommodations Network can provide you with information on available resources to help you on the job.
- Working from home can be a viable option.

Chapter 20

Patient Advocacy and Arthritis: Moving Forward

In This Chapter

- What advocacy is all about
- From 2002 to 2011: the Bone and Joint Decade
- Finding agencies that can help
- Partnering for your health
- Make your voice heard!

Patient advocacy means that people have the right to make their own choices about their health care. It assumes that to be healthy, people must be able to change their behavior and the social situations and institutions that influence their lives. Advocates operate on the local, state, national, and international levels. In this chapter, you'll learn how to become an advocate for yourself or for a loved one.

Origins of Advocacy

The concept of *advocacy* has always been part of the human experience, since the first time that someone spoke up for herself or interceded on behalf of someone else. In formal terms, we think of advocacy as part of an attorney/client relationship. Someone who is trained in the law represents someone who is not. But beginning in the twentieth century, with the advent of human rights and disability and education rights, advocacy has taken on the additional meaning of the right of every citizen to equal access to services and offerings.

def•i•ni•tion

Advocacy means pleading or arguing in defense of a cause, idea, or policy. Even today, the French word for attorney is *avocat*.

Parents are critical advocates for their children. Parents look out for their children's best interests and intercede on their behalf when necessary. Usually, as we understand the term today, advocacy involves someone with greater power, skills, or training helping someone who is in a weaker position.

The advocacy movement began in earnest back in the 1960s, when the quest for civil rights gained momentum. Not limited to securing rights for people who had been denied them based on their race or ethnicity, the movement also embraced individuals with developmental and chronic disabilities. Today, advocates represent all types of organizations, individuals, and causes—running the gamut from environmental awareness to political activism to health issues.

Arthritis is the number-one cause of disability from work, yet very few are aware of its severity. With the aging of the U.S. population, the Centers for Disease Control and Prevention estimates that the number of Americans affected by arthritis will grow from 46 million in 2008 to an alarming 76 million by 2015.

The Bone and Joint Decade

The decade from 2002 to 2011 has been designated in the United States by presidential proclamation and officially endorsed by the United Nations as the Bone and Joint Decade. Since the Decade's endorsement by United Nations Secretary-General Kofi Annan and its launch in 2000 at the World Health Organization (WHO) in Geneva, Switzerland, 60 governments and more than 1,200 patient advocacy and health professional societies have become involved. In the United States, more than 90 patient advocacy organizations, health professional societies, and academic and medical centers have come together to raise awareness, improve medical education, increase research efforts, and empower patients affected by bone and joint disorders such as arthritis.

This is important for everyone who has arthritis or any of the other musculoskeletal diseases, since this national and international endorsement has given a worldwide boost to research and funding into the causes of and the cures for these diseases, professional health-care training, and patient empowerment programs.

The Decade's mission is to improve the quality of life for people with musculoskeletal disorders worldwide. It is a framework organization through which patient groups, professional societies, governments, and industry work to raise awareness, empower patients, promote cost-effective prevention and treatment, and advance understanding through research.

The Decade involves stakeholders from various clinical disciplines, such as rheumatology, orthopedics, emergency medicine and trauma, sports medicine, physical medicine, and rehabilitation in the areas of joint diseases, osteoporosis, back and spine disorders, severe trauma to the extremities, and disabling conditions in children.

An annual international patient advocate training program brings together advocates from across the globe to learn about pressing health-care issues, develop advocacy skills, and forge partnerships that bridge national borders. The Bone and Joint Decade demonstrates that governments, health professional societies, and industry and advocate groups benefit by joining forces—the arthritis patient is the ultimate benefactor.

Agencies That Help

The millions of Americans living with arthritis and other rheumatologic conditions have pushed arthritis awareness into the forefront of the public arena and created much interest in finding a cure. Public agencies and not-for-profit agencies are stepping up to the challenge.

Taxpayer-funded agencies, along with medical organizations, such as the American College of Rheumatology, are at the forefront of patient advocacy.

The Centers for Disease Control

The Centers for Disease Control and Prevention (CDC) is an agency of the federal government. Through advocacy efforts by volunteers within the Arthritis Foundation in the 1990s, legislation was created to fund critical staff positions within the CDC to counter the rise of arthritis. In 2008, the CDC's fiscal budget for arthritis was $13 million—money dedicated to public education and arthritis public health research. The CDC, which is committed to leading strategic public health efforts to promote well-being, prevent chronic disease, and achieve health equity, is partnering with the Arthritis Foundation and other organizations to improve the quality of life for adults with arthritis and to improve people's attitudes and self-management behaviors.

To address the growing problem of arthritis, the CDC, in cooperation with the Arthritis Foundation, the Association of State and Territorial Health Officials, and 90 other organizations, has developed the *National Arthritis Action Plan: A Public Health Strategy*. Through this plan, these agencies are working to realize the first-ever arthritis-related national objectives outlined in *Healthy People 2010*. This statement of national health objectives is designed to identify the most significant preventable threats to health and to establish national goals to reduce these threats.

For more information, visit www.cdc.gov and www.healthypeople.gov.

The Arthritis Foundation

The Arthritis Foundation is the largest private, not-for-profit contributor to arthritis research in the world. Since 1948, the Foundation has funded more than $380 million in research grants. The Foundation helps people take control of their arthritis by providing public health education, pursuing public policy and legislation, and conducting evidence-based programs to improve the quality of life for those living with arthritis.

Each year, the Arthritis Foundation sponsors an Advocacy Summit in which arthritis advocates of all ages from across the country visit their representatives in person to urge them to support the Foundation's arthritis advocacy priorities. Individuals and families interested in learning how to advocate may be sponsored by their local Arthritis Foundation chapter to attend. For those who aren't able to participate in person, there is a Virtual Summit, allowing people to send e-mails to their senators and representatives, urging them to support research and legislation for arthritis. Visit www.arthritis.org for more information.

Consultation

The Arthritis Foundation has sample letters that can make corresponding with your legislators virtually painless. Check out their website at www.arthritis.org/advocacy.php.

The American College of Rheumatology

The American College of Rheumatology (ACR) is the professional society for American rheumatologists and allied health professionals. It holds an annual scientific meeting that attracts arthritis health professionals from across the globe and is the largest scientific meeting in the world. The ACR maintains a strong presence in Washington, D.C., and also helps its members with advocacy at the state and local levels.

Advocacy concerns of arthritis patients are also important to the ACR. The ACR regularly advocates for improved access to rheumatologists; more arthritis research funding; and improved insurance coverage for arthritis medications, particularly expensive new biologic therapies. During the ACR's annual Advocacy Day, members and patients go to Capitol Hill together to see members of Congress and their legislative aides and make these concerns known. For more information, visit the ACR's website at www.rheumatology.org.

National Institutes of Health

The National Institutes of Health (NIH), a part of the U.S. Department of Health and Human Services, is the primary federal agency for conducting and supporting medical research. NIH scientists investigate ways to prevent disease, as well as the causes, treatments, and even cures for common and rare diseases. Composed of 27 Institutes and Centers, the NIH provides leadership and financial support to researchers. The NIH website is www.nih.gov.

National Institute of Arthritis and Musculoskeletal and Skin Diseases

The National Institute of Arthritis and Musculoskeletal and Skin Diseases (NIAMS) was created by Congress in 1985 with a budget of $140 million. By 2002, the NIAMS budget had risen to $448.2 million.

NIAMS is part of the National Institutes of Health, an agency of the Department of Health and Human Services. Its mission is to support research into the causes, treatment, and prevention of arthritis and musculoskeletal and skin diseases, the training of basic and clinical scientists to carry out this research, and the dissemination of information on research progress in these diseases.

You can download the pamphlet "Living with Arthritis—Easy-to-Read Information for Patients and Families" from the NIAMS website. In addition to providing educational materials, NIAMS sponsors clinical trials. If you are interested in participating in one of these trials, you will find information on the website.

The Advisory Council of NIAMS consists of patient advocate leaders, along with top clinicians, researchers, and academicians. The advocates play a vital role in keeping the interests of patients and their families a central concern of the Institute. Visit www.niams.nih.gov for more information.

Specific Health Associations

In addition to the Arthritis Foundation, you are likely to find that your specific medical condition has an association. You'll find a list of these in Appendix C.

> **Straight Talk**
>
> My rheumatologist referred me to the Spondylitis Association of America. I checked out their website and decided to become a member. It was the best thing I've done to help manage AS [ankylosing spondylitis]. The support has been fantastic.
> —Jenny, age 22

These associations keep you updated on clinical trials, research grants, legislative news, recent medical advances, and other issues of concern.

The Grassroots Level

Arthritis affects everyday living at home, at work, and in the way you interact with your community. Advocating for yourself or your loved one with arthritis to get what you need is at the heart of being an effective advocate. There is a great deal that individuals can do. Many national issues also affect the individual; for example …

- Poor or delayed diagnosis of any form of arthritis.

- Delayed access from a primary-care doctor to a rheumatologist specializing in arthritis care and insufficient numbers of rheumatologists and pediatric rheumatologists to care for the growing numbers of people affected.

- Affordability of medications.

- Arthritis medications not covered or being charged higher copayments by health insurance.

- Physical and occupational therapy insufficiently covered by insurance.

- Inadequate arthritis care by primary-care providers.

- Appropriate and timely access to pediatric arthritis care.

- Access to health insurance coverage.

- Discrimination in your job due to perception of limitations from arthritis or being denied a job because of arthritis.

Advocacy at the grassroots level means personal empowerment, and there are many ways you can make your voice heard. Personal empowerment also means self-advocacy, which is the ability and commitment to speak on your own behalf. This requires that you become educated about your own diagnosis, but also that you become aware of research, pending legislation, and opportunities within your own community to get the word out.

To become a patient advocate for yourself, it's essential that you develop good communication skills and learn how to convey your concerns and questions without coming across as argumentative or difficult. Being angry or hostile does not help improve communication and may cause your health-care provider to withdraw or become defensive.

Precautions

Being a patient advocate may appear to run counter to some cultural beliefs. For example, in some Asian and Hispanic cultures, to question an elder or one of a higher educational level is considered disrespectful. It's important to understand that patient empowerment is respectful, since it guides health-care professionals to be most effective in their caregiving.

There is a need for mutual respect. For your health-care practitioner, this means recognizing that this is your body and your life. For your part, you bring your experience. You must recognize that the health-care professional (HCP) has medical expertise and is also human, just like you. Helpful tips include ...

- Find an HCP who feels right for you, one who you can openly communicate with and understand.

◆ Determine for yourself how much you want to know.

◆ Know what issues are important to you.

◆ Ask your HCP for the best time to call if you have a question.

◆ If you still have concerns, ask for a special visit to discuss the problem.

Advocating for yourself or a loved one in the medical setting is part of the movement to bring medical care back to being centered on the patient, not the practitioner. Many advocacy and medical organizations have adopted some type of a Patient's Bill of Rights. Essentially, they all agree that you have the right to ...

1. Receive answers to your health-care questions.

2. Be a fully informed participant in your health-care decisions.

3. Receive complete diagnostic information in understandable language.

4. Obtain a clear explanation of all proposed procedures, their risks and side effects, potential problems in recovery, their probability of success, and their ultimate effect on quality of life and prognosis.

5. Be able to access all information in your medical record.

6. Secure a second opinion.

7. Have your telephone calls returned.

8. Have your appointment times respected.

9. Refuse treatment or medication.

According to the philosophy expressed in the Patient's Bill of Rights, the primary function of the HCP is to prepare patients to make informed decisions about their own medical care.

Empowering the Individual

Personal advocacy enables patients with arthritis to make informed decisions about their disease and to be responsible members of their health-care teams. In order to do this, a patient must be informed about her condition and treatment options and given the opportunity to express her understandings, values, and beliefs. She must be given the time and encouragement to ask questions, raise concerns, and express her feelings about what is happening to her.

The explosive growth of the Internet has increased consumer demand for health information and has fueled the expansion of personal advocacy and disease self-management. It has become a significant tool used by advocates to inform, to mobilize grassroots attention, and to create change. However, finding reliable sources of information has become a challenge for the consumer, prompting health agencies and academic institutions to offer consumer guidelines for surfing the Internet. In some countries, direct consumer marketing by industry has resulted in higher patient demand for immediate information on medications and treatments.

Here are some tips for communicating with your health-care professional (HCP):

- Consider in advance the questions you would like to ask your HCP. Write them down.

- Take someone else along with you to the medical appointment, if you wish.

- If you wish to tape the interview, ask your HCP for permission in advance.

- Start with the most important question first; the answer you receive may change the order or nature of the other questions you wish to ask.

- Stay face to face with your HCP and ask questions in a relaxed manner. Listen carefully and note the answers.

- Ask your HCP to make a full and understandable explanation of your diagnosis and treatment, including treatment options.

- Do not make any immediate decisions regarding treatment unless you feel comfortable doing so.

- Always consider a second opinion.

Whenever we're placed in a setting that is unfamiliar or outside our comfort level, stress can build. We may sometimes confuse taking personal responsibility for our health-care management with feeling guilty for becoming ill in the first place. Sometimes this guilt may make us uncomfortable or ashamed to ask for help.

Several other issues center around personal awareness:

- We may assume health-care practitioners know what is wrong with us just by examining us; do not withhold information.

- We may feel that asking too many questions shows our ignorance.

- We may be wary of confrontation for fear of losing their respect or arousing their anger, and therefore, not receiving the best treatment or care.

Creating a healing environment is an essential component of medical care. It involves …

♦ Evaluating your needs.

♦ Normalizing your experience (this can be done effectively through mutual support or self-help groups).

♦ Giving yourself permission to experience and acknowledge your feelings.

♦ Creating ways to express your feelings about what is happening (journaling, art as therapy, talking into a tape recorder, screaming inside your car at the beach, writing poetry or songs, etc.).

Consultation

If there are usually long waiting periods at your doctor's office, call the office to see if you should arrive for your appointment later. Try to schedule the first or last appointment of the day, since this is often the best time for the least waiting.

♦ Evaluating the kind of partnership you want with your HCP.

♦ Recognizing your own biases; don't make assumptions.

♦ Gathering as much information as you wish.

♦ Remembering that you are in charge of your body and you have the most to gain by being your best advocate. This can help return some of your feelings of power and diminish feelings of loss of control.

The Patient Partner Program

The Patient Partner Program (PPP) is another example of empowerment and patient advocacy. Originally developed at the University of Texas and supported by Pharmacia and Pfizer, PPP provides training for medical students on the appropriate methods for conducting physical examinations of joints, muscles, and surrounding structures.

A unique feature of this program is that training sessions are conducted by people with arthritis who have become certified "patient partners." The patient is valued as a partner in medical teaching of arthritis.

The Chronic Disease Self-Management Program

Created by Kate Lorig, RN, and colleagues from Stanford University, the Chronic Disease Self-Management Program (CDSM) offers a comprehensive way to develop skills to manage arthritis, heart, lung, or stroke disorders. Taught by certified instructors who have a chronic disease or are health-care professionals, the program is offered two and a half hours each week for six weeks. Participants have the opportunity to partner with class members to do assignments designed to build practical knowledge and skills. Some of the topics include: techniques to deal with pain, frustration, and isolation caused by chronic disease; appropriate exercise for building strength, endurance, and flexibility; appropriate use of medications; communicating effectively with health professionals, friends, and family; the role of nutrition; and how to effectively evaluate new treatments.

The CDSM program is provided by hospitals, medical centers, and health agencies in more than 20 countries. It has proven to be effective to help participants maintain a sense of control over arthritis, better control over fatigue and pain, better communication with medical professionals, and improvements in social outreach and exercise.

The Arthritis Foundation's Arthritis Self-Help Course

Modeled after the Stanford University Chronic Disease Self-Management program, Kate Lorig, RN, and colleagues developed the Arthritis Self-Help Course (ASHC) for the Arthritis Foundation. It is regularly offered by the Arthritis Foundation in communities throughout the United States. Taught by a team of certified instructors who may have arthritis themselves, along with a health professional, the ASHC offers people affected by arthritis skills to manage their disease effectively. In two-hour sessions over six weeks, participants learn how to problem-solve for their form of arthritis; how to evaluate what exercise is appropriate for them; how to effectively communicate with their medical professionals, family, and friends; the role of nutrition and the balance of exercise; and how techniques in pain and fatigue management can help. The ASHC encourages participants to discuss and practice with class members, so interacting with them helps you help yourself while you are helping others. A foundation of the course is learning about arthritis and your needs so you can advocate effectively for yourself. Contact the Arthritis Foundation for class offerings.

The Power of Advocacy

Those who receive the best care are the ones who have mastered how to talk effectively to the people who can best help. Whether you are in a medical office, standing at the pharmacy, in school getting on a bus, or at work, how you communicate with others to get what you need can make the difference between being a victim or feeling empowered to live your life as fully as you choose.

The bottom line is that no one ever asked you if you wanted arthritis. Until there is a cure, learning all you can, becoming your own best health advocate, and partnering with your medical team have proven of be the best ways of staying active and well. And why not? We believe you're worth it.

The Least You Need to Know

♦ Advocacy groups speak out in behalf of people with disabilities, to promote research, improve access to medical care and treatments, and support legislation.

♦ The Bone and Joint Decade (2002 to 2011) endorses worldwide research and funding into the causes of and cures for arthritis, professional health-care training, and patient empowerment programs.

♦ Becoming a self-advocate can empower you to learn all you can about managing your arthritis and be a partner in your arthritis care.

♦ Joining an association that represents people with your specific diagnosis can help you stay current on important issues, treatments, and research and provide emotional and educational support as well.

♦ People working together for a common cause can accomplish nothing short of miracles.

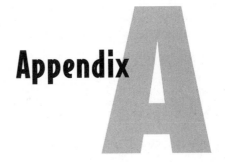

Appendix A

Glossary

acupuncture Method in traditional Chinese medicine that uses needles for therapy.

acupuncturist Person who performs acupuncture.

advanced practice nurses (APNs) Nurses who work in collaboration with physicians to provide preventative care and treatment and participate in the management of acute and chronic illnesses, such as arthritis.

advocacy Pleading or arguing in defense of a cause, idea, or policy. Even today, the French word for attorney is *avocat*.

aerobic exercise Type of exercise designed to help the heart and lungs use oxygen more efficiently.

ANA (anti-nuclear antibody) A blood test used in diagnosing lupus or other connective tissue disorders. Many people with a positive ANA have no illness at all.

analgesics Pain relievers that work by blocking the brain's reception of pain signals or by changing the way the brain interprets these signals. Analgesics can be broken into two categories: the non-narcotics and the narcotics.

anemia A condition that is defined by a low red blood cell count.

ankylosing spondylitis Type of inflammatory arthritis that affects the spine and sacroiliac joints.

anterior uveitis (iritis)   Inflammation of the front part of the uveal tract, which lines the inside of the eye behind the cornea.

antibody   Type of protein made by certain white blood cells in response to the presence of a foreign substance, called an antigen. Some antibodies help white blood cells destroy antigens, while other antibodies destroy antigens directly.

aromatherapy   Practice that uses scented essential oils to promote healing. These oils can be inhaled or used during a massage or while bathing. *See also* essential oils.

arthritis mutilans   Severe, deforming, and destructive arthritis that is associated with psoriasis.

arthritis   General term for inflammation of the joints. There are many different kinds of arthritis.

arthrocentesis   Procedure during which fluid is removed from an inflamed joint with a needle. Removing the fluid can help with diagnosis and may reduce pressure within the joint, thereby reducing pain. Medications can also be injected into the joint.

arthroplasty   Joint replacement surgery in which a severely damaged joint is repaired or replaced with an artificial one to restore function and provide pain relief.

arthroscopy   Procedure done through small incisions with special instruments that repairs or removes loose or damaged cartilage from the knee or other joints, a procedure known as debridement.

asymmetric arthritis   A type of arthritis that doesn't affect matching pairs of joints on both sides of the body.

autoantibody   An antibody formed in reaction to the body's own tissues, attacking the body it's designed to protect.

autoimmune disease   A medical condition caused by the body's immune system attacking the body it's supposed to protect.

biologic response modifiers (BRMS) or biologics   Newer class of DMARDs. These medications target very specific parts of the immune system and often provide dramatic relief of symptoms in rheumatoid arthritis and other inflammatory forms of arthritis. See also disease-modifying antirheumatic drugs (DMARDs).

body mass index (BMI)   Scale that relates your weight to your height. Your BMI is your weight in kilograms (kg) divided by your height in meters (m) squared. This tool correlates strongly with total body fat content in adults.

botanical   A plant or a plant part that's valued for its medicinal or therapeutic properties, flavor, and/or scent. Products made from botanicals may be marketed as herbal products, botanical products, or phytomedicines.

bursa   Sac filled with lubricating fluid, located at pressure points like the elbow or between tissues such as bone, muscle, tendons, and skin.

bursitis   Inflammation of the bursa.

cardiologist   Doctor specializing in diseases involving the heart.

cartilage   Firm, rubbery material covering the ends of bones in normal joints. The main function of cartilage is to reduce friction in the joints and serve as a shock absorber.

central nervous system   A system that consists of the brain and spinal cord.

chiropractic   Literally meaning "done by hand," the ancient practice of manipulation to the spine as a means of healing.

chondroitin   A normal component of cartilage and also a nutritional supplement.

chronic illness   Ongoing and long-term illness.

clinical trials   Tests designed to evaluate the effectiveness and safety of medications or medical devices through the monitoring of their effects on large groups of people.

CMC (first carpometacarpal) joint   Where the thumb joint connects with the wrist.

corticosteroids   *See* steroids.

cortisone   Potent anti-inflammatory corticosteroid.

COX-2 inhibitors   Newer type of nonsteroidal anti-inflammatory drug (NSAID) that relieves inflammation. *See also* nonsteroidal anti-inflammatory drugs (NSAIDs).

CPAP   Continuous positive airway pressure. A CPAP device, used to treat sleep apnea, is worn on your face and secured with straps around your head.

C-reactive protein (CRP)   Protein found in the blood that indicates the amount of inflammation present within the body.

culture   Process of cultivating microorganisms in a growth medium. It's done in a medical laboratory. Any body tissue or fluid can be evaluated in a laboratory by this method to detect and identify infectious agents.

degenerative joint disease   *See* osteoarthritis.

DEXA scan   Imaging test to determine bone density. Low bone density is an indicator of osteoporosis.

DIP (distal interphalangeal) joint   First joint below the fingertips.

disease-modifying antirheumatic drugs (DMARDs)   Prescription medications that slow or halt the progress of rheumatoid and other inflammatory forms of arthritis.

endorphins   Chemicals produced by the body during times of pain or stress. Endorphins relieve pain.

enteropathic arthritis   A form of chronic, inflammatory arthritis that is associated with the occurrence of inflammatory bowel disease (IBD).

enzyme   Protein that acts as a catalyst to speed up the body's biochemical reactions. The most important enzymes for treating inflammation are collectively called the proteases.

erythrocyte sedimentation rate (ESR or sed rate)   Blood test that can indicate the degree of inflammation in the body.

fascia   A thin layer of connective tissue that covers or connects the muscles or inner organs of the body.

flare   A period of increased disease activity.

glandulars   Extracts of animal organs, containing hormones and other substances contained within those organs.

glucosamine   A building block of cartilage and a nutritional supplement.

gout   Type of crystalline arthritis caused by a buildup of uric acid crystals in the joints.

HLA-B27   Cell surface protein found on white blood cells associated with a gene linked to ankylosing spondylitis.

homeopathy   Alternative medicine practice operating on the principle that "like cures like."

hyaluronic acid   Substance occurring naturally in the joint fluid that acts as a lubricant and cushion for the knee joint. It may also have anti-inflammatory and pain-relieving properties.

hydrotherapy   Therapy using water.

immune system   The body's defense system against infectious and other diseases.

inflammation   Process occurring when the body's white blood cells and chemicals mobilize to protect the body against infection and foreign substances (such as bacteria and viruses). Inflammation is characterized by redness, warmth, swelling, and pain. Inflammation is a symptom of autoimmune and crystalline diseases.

insomnia   Literally meaning "without sleep," this refers both to a difficulty in falling asleep and difficulty in staying asleep.

iridocyclitis   Inflammation of the iris and the ciliary body—two structures within the front part of the eye.

isometrics   *See* strengthening exercises.

isotonics   Exercises that use repetitions or light resistance to increase joint mobility.

joint aspiration   Procedure that removes some fluid from a joint. The fluid may be sent to a medical lab for analysis.

joint contracture   Limited range of motion of a joint caused by shortening of the muscles or tendons that surround the joint.

joint replacement surgery   Surgical procedure to replace natural joints with synthetic ones to restore function.

joint   Location where two bones meet.

juvenile arthritis (JA)   The most common form of arthritis affecting children. Also called juvenile inflammatory arthritis (JIA) and, previously, juvenile rheumatoid arthritis (JRA).

ligament   Structure that connects bones and keeps joints stable.

longitudinal studies   Research studies that follow the same people over an extended period of time.

low-level laser therapy (LLLT)   An alternative medicine technique using a light source that's believed by some to generate photochemical reactions within the body's cells to decrease pain and swelling.

lupus   *See* systemic lupus erythematosus (SLE).

Lyme disease   Spirochete infection that is transmitted by a tick bite.

magnetic resonance imaging (MRI)   Test that uses a large magnet, electromagnetic energy waves, and a computer to produce images.

mantra   Sound used in meditation. Reciting your mantra removes all outside distractions and encourages you to relax and become at peace.

metabolic syndrome (syndrome X)   Cluster of risk factors that increase risk of cardiovascular disease. These factors include insulin resistance (diabetes), high blood pressure, cholesterol abnormalities, and large waist size (abdominal obesity).

metabolites   Any of the substances produced by the metabolism—the entire range of biochemical processes occurring within the body.

methylsulfonylmethane (MSM)   Naturally occurring sulfur-containing chemical sometimes used as a dietary supplement.

narcotic   A drug that reduces pain, alters mood or behavior, and usually induces sleep or stupor. Narcotics are stronger pain relievers than analgesics but also have the potential to be addicting.

nephrologist   Doctor specializing in treating kidney disease.

neurologist   Doctor specializing in disorders of the nervous system.

neurotransmitters   Chemicals carrying nerve impulses between nerve fibers.

nonsteroidal anti-inflammatory drugs (NSAIDs)   A class of medicines known to reduce inflammation and relieve pain.

occupational therapy   Therapy that provides help with managing everyday activities.

ophthalmologist   Doctor specializing in treating diseases of the eye.

osteoarthritis   The most common type of arthritis. Also called degenerative joint disease.

osteophyte   Bone spur that forms as the result of changes caused by osteoarthritis.

osteoporosis   Condition that causes loss of bone tissue, leading to increased risk of fractures.

osteotomy   Surgery to realign the bones.

parvovirus   A virus that can cause infectious arthritis in children or adults.

pauciarticular juvenile arthritis   Type of juvenile arthritis involving up to four joints.

pericarditis   An inflammation of the membrane located around the heart.

phototherapy   Therapy using natural or artificial light.

physical therapy   Program of exercise and other treatments to help keep your muscles strong and your joints from becoming stiff.

physician assistant   A health-care practitioner who works under the supervision of a physician.

PIP (proximal interphalangeal) joint   The middle joint on the finger.

placebo   Inactive substance used in clinical trials.

podiatrist   Physician who specializes in evaluating and treating diseases of the foot.

polyarticular juvenile arthritis   Type of juvenile arthritis involving five or more joints.

prolotherapy   A controversial therapy involving injection of a sugar solution into the soft tissues around joints to cause stiffening and stability.

prostaglandins   Body chemicals that help send pain messages to the brain and also promote inflammation and fever, support the function of platelets necessary for blood to clot, and protect the stomach from acidic damage.

pseudogout   Form of crystalline arthritis caused by a buildup of calcium pyrophosphate crystals in the joints.

psoriasis   Inflammatory skin disorder characterized by redness and itching; thick, dry, silvery scales; and nail abnormalities.

psoriatic arthritis   Form of inflammatory arthritis that affects some people with psoriasis.

purine   White crystalline substance that's one of the building blocks of DNA. When purine is broken down in the body as part of the metabolic process, it creates uric acid.

range of motion   The normal distance a joint can move.

range of motion exercises   Exercises designed to maintain or increase normal joint function.

reactive arthritis   Condition that develops as the result of certain infections. It affects the spine and the sacroiliac joints (the area where the spine attaches to the pelvis). It can also affect various other joints of the body, including the arms and legs. Reactive arthritis used to be called Reiter's Syndrome.

resistance exercises   *See* strengthening exercises.

restless legs syndrome (RLS)   The unrelenting urge to move your legs to relieve an overwhelming unpleasant sensation.

revision arthroplasty   A second surgery that's required to replace a joint replacement that has worn out or failed.

Reye's Syndrome   A rare disease that may occur in children with the flu or chicken pox who are also taking aspirin.

rheumatic disease   Disease that causes inflammation or degeneration in the body's connective tissues, especially the joints (the places where two or more bones meet).

rheumatoid arthritis   A type of chronic inflammatory arthritis.

rheumatoid factor   Variety of antibodies present in 70 to 90 percent of people with rheumatoid arthritis.

rheumatologist   Physician specialist who treats arthritis, certain immune system diseases, and osteoporosis.

SAM-e   Synthetic form of a byproduct of an amino acid that occurs naturally in the human body and helps produce hormones and cell membranes. Promoted as a dietary supplement for arthritis but with very little scientific evidence.

scleroderma   Rheumatologic condition involving overproduction of collagen, the protein that's the building block for bone, cartilage, tendons, and other connective tissues.

Sjögren's syndrome   Chronic disorder that causes insufficient moisture production.

skeletal maturity   When bones meet skeletal maturity, they have achieved maximum growth. A doctor uses X-ray imagery of the bones to discover their developmental stage and determine whether skeletal maturity has been reached.

sleep apnea   A sometimes serious and potentially life-threatening condition in which an individual stops breathing repeatedly during sleep, sometimes hundreds of times during the night and occasionally for a minute or longer.

slit-lamp eye examination   Examination that uses magnified three-dimensional imagery to view the different parts of the eye.

spirochete   A spiral-shaped microscopic organism.

spondylitis   Type of arthritis affecting the spinal column and sacroiliac joints.

spondyloarthropies   Arthritic conditions affecting the spinal joints, ligaments, and tendons.

steroids   Synthetic drugs given either orally or by injection and used to treat a variety of inflammatory diseases and conditions.

strengthening exercises   Also known as resistance exercises. They build the muscles that support your joints.

stressor   Anything that upsets the balance of physical reactions in your body. Your reaction to stress is to a large extent a function of your personality, general health, physical strength, and psychological well-being.

supportive (assistive) devices   Devices used to assist with the activities of daily living.

synovectomy   Removal of an inflamed joint lining (synovium).

synovial fluid   The fluid found within joints.

synovium   The lining of a joint.

systemic juvenile arthritis   Type of juvenile arthritis that affects both the joints and the internal organs.

systemic lupus erythematosus (SLE)   Often referred to simply as lupus. A chronic inflammatory autoimmune disease affecting the joints, kidneys, lungs, nervous system, skin, and other organs of the body.

target heart rate   Term for the optimum pulse rate you reach during exercise, when your circulatory system is working at full efficiency.

tendinitis   Inflammation of a tendon.

tendon   Thick tissue cord that attaches bone to muscle.

TENS   Transcutaneous electrical nerve stimulation. A small device that directs mild electrical impulses to nerves in the painful joint or muscle area. These nerve impulses work to block pain signals and may also release endorphins.

tophi   Gritty nodules that form just under the skin or in joints in people with gout, caused by an accumulation of uric acid crystals.

uric acid   Substance found in urine.

vasculitis   Inflammation of blood vessels, including veins and arteries.

vertebrae   Bones of the spine.

viscosupplementation   Procedure in which hyaluronic acid derivatives are injected into an osteoarthritic joint.

yoga   Discipline from ancient India that unites mind, body, and spirit.

Appendix B

Acronyms

AC acromioclavicular joint

ADA Americans with Disabilities Act

AMA American Medical Association

AMTA American Massage Therapy Association

AS ankylosing spondylitis

ASA acetylsalicylic acid

BMI body mass index

BRMs biologic response modifiers

CAM complementary and alternative medicine

CDC Centers for Disease Control

CMC carpometacarpal joint

DEA Drug Enforcement Agency

DIP distal interphalangeal joint

DMARDs disease-modifying antirheumatic drugs

EA enteropathic arthritis

EEOC Equal Employment Opportunity Commission

ESR erythrocyte sedimentation rate (sed rate)

FDA Food and Drug Administration

FMLA Family and Medical Leave Act

HAL-2 Handicapped Assistance Loan

HDL high-density lipoprotein

IBD inflammatory bowel disease

IDEA Individuals with Disabilities Education Act

IEP Individualized Education Program

JA juvenile arthritis

JAMA *Journal of the American Medical Association*

JAN Job Accommodation Network

JIA juvenile idiopathic arthritis

JRA juvenile rheumatoid arthritis

LDL low-density lipoprotein

LLLT low-level laser therapy

MAMDC Multipurpose Arthritis and Musculoskeletal Diseases Center

MSM methylsulfonylmethane

NCCAM National Center for Complementary and Alternative Medicine

NIAMS National Institute of Arthritis and Musculoskeletal and Skin Diseases

NIH National Institutes of Health

NSAIDs nonsteroidal anti-inflammatory drugs

OA osteoarthritis

ODEP Office of Disability Employment Policy

OT occupational therapy/occupational therapist

OTC over-the-counter (medication)

PIP proximal interphalangeal joint

PT   physical therapy/physical therapist

RA   rheumatoid arthritis

RF   rheumatoid factor

RSA   Rehabilitation Services Administration

SAM-e   S-adenosylmethionine

SBA   Small Business Administration

SLE   systemic lupus erythematosus (lupus)

SNRIs   serotonin-norepinephrine reuptake inhibitors (dual inhibitors)

SSDI   Social Security Disability Insurance

SSI   Supplemental Security Income

TENS   transcutaneous nerve stimulation

TNF   tumor necrosis factor (blockers)

Appendix **C**

Resources

American Academy of Orthopaedic Surgeons
6300 North River Road
Rosemont, IL 60018-4262
1-800-346-AAOS (346-2267)
www.aaos.org

Information on orthopaedic conditions and treatments, injury prevention,
wellness and exercise, and more.

American Autoimmune Related Diseases Association
22100 Gratiot Avenue
East Detroit, MI 48021-2227
1-800-598-4668
aarda@aarda.org
www.aarda.org

The only national nonprofit health agency dedicated to bringing a national
focus to autoimmunity, the major cause of serious chronic diseases.

American College of Rheumatology
1800 Century Place, Suite 250
Atlanta, GA 30345-4300
www.rheumatology.org

An organization of and for physicians, health professionals, and scientists that advances rheumatology through programs of education, research, advocacy, and practice support that foster excellence in the care of people with arthritis and rheumatic and musculoskeletal diseases.

Arthritis Foundation
P.O. Box 7669
Atlanta, GA 30357-0669
1-800-283-7800
www.arthritis.org

A not-for-profit organization that supports different types of arthritis and related conditions with advocacy, programs, services, and research.

Job Accommodation Network (JAN)
West Virginia University
P.O. Box 6080
Morgantown, WV 26506-6080
1-800-526-7234
TTY: 1-877-781-9403
www.jan.wvu.edu

A free consulting service that provides information about job accommodations, the Americans with Disabilities Act (ADA), and the employability of people with disabilities.

Missouri Arthritis Rehabilitation Research and Training Center
Missouri School of Journalism
Walter Williams Hall, Room 13
Columbia, MO 65211
1-877-882-6826
marrtc@missouri.edu
marrtc.missouri.edu

The only federally funded arthritis rehabilitation research and training center in the country.

National Center for Complementary and Alternative Medicine (NCCAM)
9000 Rockville Pike
Bethesda, MD 20892
1-888-644-6226
info@nccam.nih.gov
nccam.nih.gov

The federal government's lead agency for scientific research on complementary and alternative medicine (CAM) and 1 of the 27 institutes and centers that make up the National Institutes of Health (NIH) within the U.S. Department of Health and Human Services.

National Institute of Arthritis and Musculoskeletal and Skin Diseases
1 AMS Circle
Bethesda, MD 20892-3675
1-877-22N-IAMS (226-4267)
TTY: 301-565-2966
niamsinfo@mail.nih.gov
www.niams.nih.gov

Supports research into the causes, treatment, and prevention of arthritis and musculoskeletal and skin diseases, the training of basic and clinical scientists to carry out this research, and the dissemination of information on research progress in these diseases.

National Institutes of Health (NIH)
9000 Rockville Pike
Bethesda, MD 20892
www.nih.gov

Part of the U.S. Department of Health and Human Services and the primary federal agency for conducting and supporting medical research.

Office of Disability Employment Policy (ODEP)
200 Constitution Avenue, NW, Room S-1303
Washington, D.C. 20210
202-693-7880
TTY: 202-693-7881
infoODEP@dol.gov
www.dol.gov/odep/

Provides national leadership on disability employment policy by developing and influencing the use of evidence-based disability employment policies and practices, building collaborative partnerships, and delivering authoritative and credible data on employment of people with disabilities.

Spondylitis Association of America
P.O. Box 5872
Sherman Oaks, CA 91413
1-800-777-8189
info@spondylitis.org
www.spondylitis.org

Their mission is "to be a leader in the quest to cure ankylosing spondylitis and related diseases and to empower those affected to live life to the fullest."

Index

B

N

Check out these BEST-SELLERS

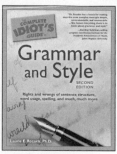

Grammar and Style SECOND EDITION

Rights and wrongs of sentence structure, word usage, spelling, and much, much more

Laurie E. Rozakis, Ph.D.

978-1-59257-115-4
$16.95

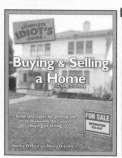

Buying & Selling a Home FIFTH EDITION

Solid strategies for getting the best deal—whether you're buying or selling

Shelley O'Hara and Nancy D. Lewis

978-1-59257-458-2
$19.95

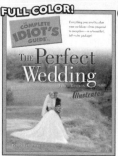

FULL COLOR!

THE **Perfect Wedding** *Illustrated*

978-1-59257-566-4
$22.95

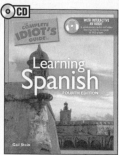

CD

Learning Spanish FOURTH EDITION

Gail Stein

978-1-59257-485-8
$24.95

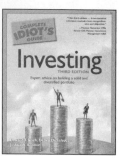

Investing THIRD EDITION

Expert advice on building a solid and diversified portfolio

978-1-59257-480-3

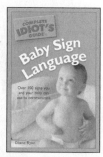

Baby Sign Language

Over 100 signs you and your baby can use to communicate

Diane Ryan

978-1-59257-469-8
$14.95

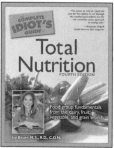

Total Nutrition FOURTH EDITION

Food group fundamentals from the dairy, fruit, vegetable, and grain worlds

Joy Bauer, M.S., R.D., C.D.N.

978-1-59257-439-1
$18.95

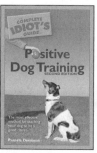

Positive Dog Training SECOND EDITION

The most effective method for teaching your dog to be a good citizen

Pamela Dennison

978-1-59257-483-4
$14.95

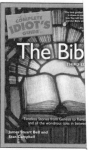

The Bible THIRD EDITION

Timeless Stories from Genesis to Revelation and all the wondrous tales in between

James Stuart Bell and Stan Campbell

978-1-59257-389-9
$18.95

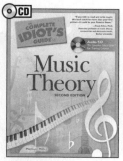

CD

Music Theory SECOND EDITION

Michael Miller

978-1-59257-437-7
$19.95

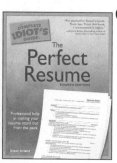

The Perfect Resume FOURTH EDITION

Professional help in making your resume stand out from the pack

Susan Ireland

978-1-59257-463-6
$14.95

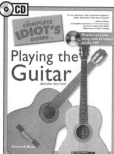

CD

Playing the Guitar SECOND EDITION

Frederick Noad

978-0-02864244-4
$21.95

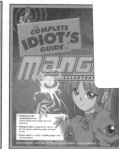

Manga *Illustrated*

John Layman and David Macho Gonzales

978-1-59257-335-6
$19.95

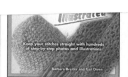

Illustrated

Keep your stitches straight with hundreds of step-by-step photos and illustrations

Barbara Breiter and Gail Diven

978-1-59257-491-9
$19.95

More than **450 titles** available at booksellers and online retailers everywhere

ALPHA
www.idiotsguides.com